# Self-Massage
# for
# **Athletes**

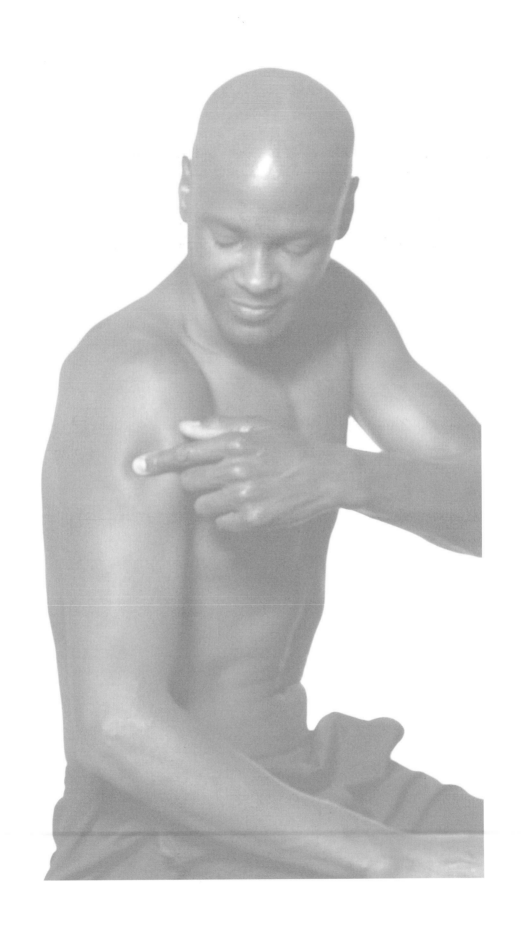

# Self-Massage For Athletes

The Hands-On Guide
To Improve Your
Athletic Performance,
Relieve Your Aches and Pains,
and Help You Feel Better Fast

Rich Poley

Two Hand Press, LLC
Boulder, Colorado

# Self-Massage for Athletes
Rich Poley

Two Hand Press, LLC, P.O. Box 4236, Boulder, Colorado 80306
© 2006 by Rich Poley.
All rights reserved. Published 2006
14 13 12 11 10 09 08 07 06    1 2 3 4 5

ISBN:-10: 0-9776086-0-3
ISBN:-13: 978-0-9776086-0-7

Editor: Ellen Orleans

Grateful acknowledgment is made to Doubleday for permission to reprint an excerpt from page 51 of *My Life and the Beautiful Game*, by Pelé with Robert L. Fish, 1977.
Grateful acknowledgment is made to Houghton Mifflin Company for permission to reprint excerpts from pages 58, 61, 96–97 of *Health and Healing*, by Andrew Weil, M.D., © 1995 by Andrew Weil.

LCCN: 2005910636

Self-Massage for Athletes: The Hands-On Guide to Improve Your Athletic Performance, Relieve Your Aches and Pains, and Help You Feel Better Fast

Visit www.SelfMassageForAthletes.com for additional information, massage tools, and links to Web sites relating to self-massage.

**Printed in the United States of America**

# Acknowledgments

To the many athletes who attended my early workshops at Fleet Feet Sports in Boulder, Colorado: Thanks for teaching me how to teach self-massage.

To **Kathy Hawk Boyd,** thanks for all your help, encouragement, and support. You are the greatest.

To **Gina Simmering-Lanterman** and **Dyrone Minors**, thank you for your friendship, support, and help whenever I need it, which is always.

To all who read and edited early drafts of this book, a heartfelt thanks, especially to **Elizabeth Wells, Steve Foster, Tom Rafferty, Neal Henderson, Phil Astrachan, Dr. Yun Tao Ma, Dr. Jamie Foster, Win Johnson, Jack Kerner, Dr. Leonard Shlain, Holly Terry, Leah Garcia,** and **Tracey Holderman.**

To everyone I bothered, pestered, and begged to read this, look at that, and try this, especially to **Elizabeth Guare, Steve Alpert, Jim Pruett, Everett James Gonzales, Marco Coelho, Mikalle Higby, Roberto Bianco, Jen Fisher, Lizzie Davis, Daphne McCabe, Rick Ellison, Larry Poley, Mike Ricci, Carrie Thigpen, Susan Wilson, Carl Kinney, Adam Chase, Nicole Deboom, Jane Scott, Dave Scott, Chuckie V., Cisco Quintero, Laurie Edwards, Todd Straka, KC, Stephen Pifer, Michael Lovato, Maria Uspenski, Colleen Schreiner, Scott Fliegelman, Greg Cunningham, Lilly Guerra Johnson, Jay Johnson, Vicki Hunter, Nancy Kauffold, Tia Boddington, Mary Foley, Lolita Bryan, Lynne Epple, Jan Ward,** and **Michael Levy.**

To all the athletes who were interviewed for this book, and to everyone who contributed to this book, your generosity will be appreciated by all who learn from it.

# Covers

Athletes whose color photos appear on the covers of this book are **Erin Kummer, Scott Fliegelman, Melody Fairchild, Adam Chase, Elizabeth Wells, Mike Ricci, Barry Siff, Marco Coelho,** and **Gina Simmering-Lanterman.**

*He who knows others is wise;*
*he who knows himself is enlightened.*
—Lao Tzu

*No matter how simple the task, if it's broken up into*
*enough of its component parts it will soon become impossible.*

# CONTENTS

# PART II: Learning Self-Massage

# PART III: Going Deeper: Getting More from Your Massage

# Table of Athletes in Action

Many of the athletes photographed in this book are identified here along with their photographer. All other black and white photos appearing on these pages are by Tim Benko of Benko Photographics.

# PART I

# Why Every Athlete Needs Massage

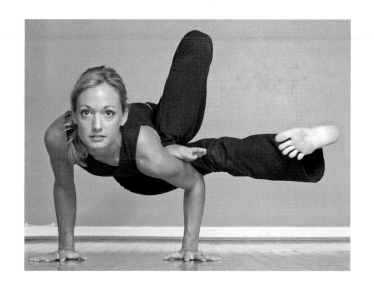

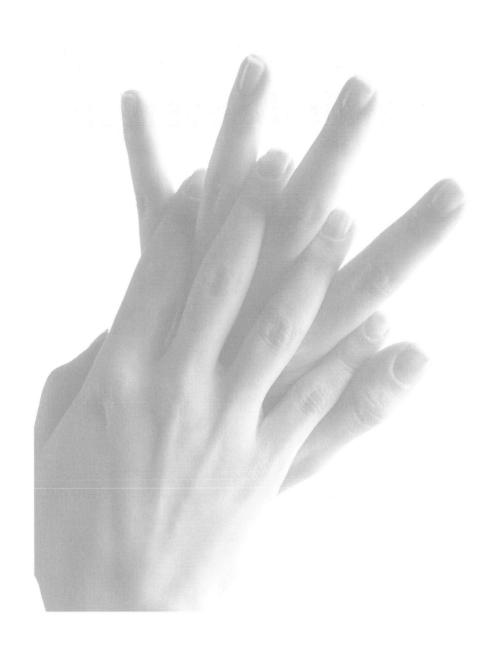

# 1

# Your Introduction to Self-Massage

## How This Book Can Help You

If you've ever used your own hands to work out a kink in your calf, soothe a pain in your shoulder, or relieve a cramp in your foot, this book is for you. In these pages you'll find many exciting ways to help you reach your athletic goals and to improve your fitness, health, and mood. You'll find massage techniques and tips that you won't find anyplace else.

If you're an athlete and want to relieve sore muscles after a workout, reduce recovery time, decrease your chances of getting injured, gain a new understanding of your body, or simply relieve tension and relax, this book is for you. Whether you're trying self-massage for the first time or are a veteran looking for new ideas, this book will help you achieve your goals. Even if you just want to learn to give someone else a massage, this book will help you. The easiest way to learn to massage others is to learn what works best on you; this book provides you with the tools to do just that.

*Self-Massage for Athletes* was written for recreational and professional athletes alike. It doesn't matter what sports you play or activities you do. It doesn't matter whether your sport of choice is running, yoga, golf, cycling, swimming, Pilates, blading, boxing, skiing, wrestling, pitching horseshoes or baseballs, lifting weights, dancing, playing football, jumping out of airplanes, or twirling hoola-hoops. You may not even consider yourself an athlete. But if you regularly and vigorously use your body, in the pursuit of fitness, pleasure, or excellence, you're an athlete. The Surgeon General of the United States says about thirty million Americans fit the definition of an athlete.

Let's face it, everyone needs a massage after a hard workout. Until now, the cost and time it took to get one left that need unmet. This book changes that. It removes the recurring costs and makes massage accessible to everybody. Even if you see a massage therapist regularly, self-massage can help you fine-tune your sessions and become a co-creator with your therapist.

As an athlete, if your muscles get sore, self-massage can fix you right up. With massage, muscle pain disappears. It's gone like that, the way your fist vanishes when you open your hand.

Many of us are uncomfortable touching our own bodies. As a matter of fact, the only people who seem entirely comfortable with their bodies are professional baseball players.* If you're uncomfortable with your body, this book will help you get over that feeling and get back in touch with yourself.

The techniques described in these pages apply to anyone who wants to feel better. If you've ever suffered muscle soreness, you'll find the ideas, advice, and instructions in this book apply to you. All the massage strokes work equally well for athletes and non-athletes. Because athletes have developed their bodies to a greater extent than others, they'll notice more benefits.

## Advantages of Self-Massage

While many of the benefits self-massage offers are identical to those you would receive from a professional massage therapist, self-massage also provides a unique set of benefits. To get the most significant health benefits, clinical research shows that massage should be received at least twice a week.[1] The cost of a professional massage twice a week puts these health benefits out of reach for most people. With self-massage, these health benefits are within everyone's reach. In fact, they're never farther away than your own fingertips.

Another advantage of self-massage is perfect feedback. With self-massage, the person giving the massage is the person getting the massage. So the person giving the massage gets immediate feedback on the effect of each stroke. That's one reason self-massage may be more effective than other forms of massage.

A third advantage of self-massage is immediacy. With self-massage, you receive the benefits when you most need them. No need to make an appointment with a therapist or beg a friend or

---

*To their credit, baseball players can be seen continually massaging themselves during games. They have special coaches stationed along the first and third base lines who, while moving their hands over their bodies, appear to use self-massage to communicate with their players.

loved one. Self-massage also gives you an understanding of your body that you can't get from anyone else.

That said, self-massage is not intended to entirely replace other forms of massage. It won't replace massage therapy for treating injuries or for deep tissue work. It may, however, be used in concert with a massage therapist's guidance for treating injuries. It also will not replace the spa massage. While self-massage can be relaxing, it will not produce the feeling of total pampering people report from a spa massage. It won't replace the connection people feel when a friend or loved one touches them. But self-massage will give you the power to make yourself feel better anytime and anywhere you like.

## My Story

I first learned what an amazing tool self-massage could be for athletes while training for my first Ironman distance triathlon. My training was going badly. I'd wake up every morning sore and weak. I knew that professional athletes used massage and self-massage to help them train. So I took up self-massage to help me train more effectively. And it worked. Not only was my muscle soreness gone, but I recovered faster from my training. I also noticed an improvement in my mood and health. I felt great. With self-massage, completing my first big triathlon was fun and easy.

I've spent more than forty years as a recreational athlete and clocked thousands of hours training for all kinds of sports: from golf to skydiving, yoga to basketball. I first learned self-massage to heal my own aching muscles. I had no special knowledge of anatomy or medical training, which proves that you don't need medical expertise to learn to massage your own body. Since learning self-massage, I've taught hundreds of recreational athletes self-massage and, with their help, I learned how to effectively teach self-massage. The book you are holding in your hand is unique. At this writing, no other book teaches self-massage to athletes, gives you a better understanding of its benefits, or offers an easier way to learn its techniques.

## What You'll Learn

The following pages show you how to effectively use self-massage. You'll learn a simple system that will guide you stroke by stroke until you are able to guide yourself. You won't need massage oils, special equipment, or expert knowledge of human anatomy. All you'll need are your hands, your body, this book, and a desire to feel better.

In **Part I** of the book, you'll learn how self-massage improves your health, mood, and athletic performance. You'll learn why massage makes you feel better and how you can use it to reach your athletic goals. You'll learn how to activate your endorphin delivery system. You'll discover some of the mysteries of your own body and how it absorbs the enormous benefits of massage.

In **Part II**, you'll learn the *seven simple massage strokes* that make up a great massage. You'll learn by doing each one as you read. Then you'll put the strokes together while learning to massage your entire body. You'll learn to improvise and invent stroke combinations to meet your changing needs. By the time you've finished this part of the book, you'll know how to perform a full body massage and will have the power to make yourself feel better anytime you want.

In **Part III**, you'll learn to go deeper into massage. You'll learn ways to improve your massage. You'll learn how to fine-tune your massage by exploring the secrets of acupressure, trigger point therapy, shower massage, and some potent massage tools. You'll explore new techniques and learn about yourself in a whole new way.

When you finish this book, you will have all the skills you need to give yourself a great massage anytime you want.

## In Summary

As an athlete, you can do more for your body than you realize. You can improve your health, relieve your pain, reduce your chances of injury, and increase your athletic performance through a regular practice of self-massage.

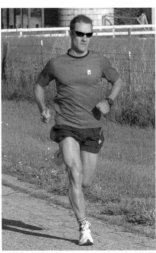

# 2

# Advantages of Self-Massage

## Why Self-Massage May Be the Best Kind of Massage

While this chapter describes the powerful benefits of self-massage, we're not suggesting that self-massage is better than other forms of massage. Nor are we saying that self-massage is more effective than massage therapy for treating injuries. In fact, few things feel better than putting yourself in the hands of a skilled massage therapist to relieve injuries and sore muscles or relax. Getting a friend or loved one to massage your aches and pains can also be wonderful, while going to a spa for a full body massage may be the most relaxing thing you can do for yourself. We're certainly not knocking any of these alternatives to self-massage.

Because this is a book advocating self-massage, however, it's appropriate to discuss the advantages and even some of the disadvantages of self-massage. Let's start out by identifying some of the advantages.

- **Learn It Fast:** Self-massage is easy to learn because it's essentially instinctive.

- **Learning About Yourself**: Self-massage is the quintessential hands-on learning experience in which you're the student, teacher, and subject.

- **Cost**: Self-massage is affordable.

- **Self-Empowering**: With self-massage, you're empowering

yourself to relieve muscle pain, speed recovery, improve health, and feel better fast. You don't have to plan your schedule around someone else's. Not even the closest friend is always within touching distance. Plus, self-massage eliminates the need for begging and groveling; you'll never have to beg a friend or loved one for a massage again.

- **Availability**: Self-massage is accessible anywhere.

- **Immediacy**: Self-massage is accessible immediately, even right after workouts when finding someone to touch you, even if you pay them, may be impossible.

- **Dual Benefit**: With self-massage, you get two massages every time you perform one.

- **Massaging Others**: If you want to learn to massage another person, self-massage is one of the easiest, most effective ways to learn.

- **Frequency**: Many of the major health benefits produced by massage—including improved immune system function, reduced stress, anxiety, and depression—only occur with frequent massage, two or more times a week: More about this in Chapter 3.

There are, of course, disadvantages to self-massage. Chief among them is that it's difficult to effectively self-treat an injury. When injured, you should consult a healthcare professional. Depending on the injury, a massage therapist may be a good place to start. Even if you are a healthcare professional, getting a second opinion is important. After consulting a trusted professional, you may use self-massage in concert with the professional to help heal yourself.

A second disadvantage of self-massage is that you can't relax as fully as you can when another set of hands is giving the massage. A third disadvantage of self-massage is reach; it's hard to reach your back—but this is a problem with a simple solution.

## The Next Big Thing

The rest of this chapter is devoted to exploring some of these advantages and disadvantages of self-massage. A special focus will be to discover why self-massage is the most often used and under-used therapy in sports today, and why it's likely to become the next big thing in sports medicine.

## Easy to Learn

With so many benefits of self-massage, it's surprising that athletes have not taken more advantage of them. After all, self-massage is easy to learn. There are only three basic moves: (1) gliding, (2) pressing, and (3) pulling. It's practically instinctive. Every mammal does it. If they don't have hands, they use paws, tongues, or rub up against trees or the earth. Every human being uses self-massage. Most of the time, we're not even aware we're massaging ourselves because it comes so naturally to us.

Still, there are specific techniques that make self-massage much more effective. While well known to professional massage therapists, these simple techniques are largely unknown outside the profession. Athletes tend to learn self-massage quickly and use it effectively when they're shown these techniques.

## Why It's Easy to Learn

If you believe it takes a skilled massage therapist with a highly trained sense of touch to perform an effective massage, you're in good company. Many athletes believe that. As you'll learn, though, self-massage requires very little training, and a sense of touch that you already possess. It's been observed that self-massage is an almost perfect information system, a kind of self-healing feedback loop. Think of your body and mind as an information system. When you use self-massage, you get immediate information about how each stroke feels. This immediate feedback directs your next stroke. It tells you where it should be, how hard it should be, and what kind of stroke it should be.

Adam Chase, attorney, father, and coauthor of *The Ultimate Guide to Trail Running,* uses self-massage to keep warm and improve circulation during long adventure races that often last days. He says, "Touch is fairly healing. Because you are in your own body, only you really know exactly how hard to push, how deep is okay, what might be injurious, what feels best. A really good massage therapist, especially someone who is an athlete might have some insight, but they're not in your body. They can't feel inside of you, and that is what puts self-massage at such a premium." Adam has no formal training in massage. He says, "it's something that's easy to learn and natural for athletes to do."

## Learning about Yourself

Ultimately, self-massage is a way of exploring yourself. It teaches you about your body in a way anatomy books and doctors cannot. You learn to understand your own aches and pains, how to access trigger points, activate acupoints, and release endorphins. After all, self-massage is the origin of massage therapy, acupressure, and acupuncture.

What you learn about yourself will help you train more effectively. Getting more in touch with your body will help you feel its strengths and weaknesses, will let you know when to train hard, and when to stay home, thus reducing your likelihood of injury.

Head triathlon coach Mike Ricci says, "Whenever I have an ache or pain, I work on that area until I have reduced the pain and I feel as though it won't be a hindrance the next day. I tend to know my body pretty well, but the self-massage techniques I've learned come in very handy!"

## Custom Massage

One advantage of self-massage is that it allows you to custom fit your massage to your changing needs while helping you discover a pattern of massage to meet your own overall needs. For instance, your needs may change with the season as you move from skiing to swimming, or as you move from high intensity training to tapering before a big race. In addition, because you know your own body, you are aware of its special needs.

Sunny Gilbert, triathlete and former coach of the national championship University of Colorado triathlon team, says, "I massage sore spots almost as soon as they pop up. For me, self-massage is an anytime, anywhere occurrence that helps me relieve physical and mental stress. I know I dig into my foot (plantar fasciitis) almost every night. And when I was coming back from my car accident and building up my shoulder strength again for swimming, I had to work out knots just about every session as different muscles came on-line at their own rate. I went from total shoulder freeze to swimming over 1,000 yards per session in just about six weeks that way."

## Cost-Benefit Analysis

Most athletes believe that the key benefit of self-massage is that it's free. But that's not a benefit as much as it is a quality. The cost of self-massage has no real significance until you analyze its many benefits. After all, a sprained ankle is free but it provides few benefits. Here's a simple analysis showing the benefits of self-massage relative to their costs.

| Benefits of Self-Massage | Costs of Self-Massage |
|---|---|
| Relieves Muscle Pain | $ 0.00 |
| Speeds Recovery | $ 0.00 |
| Reduces Likelihood of Injury | $ 0.00 |
| Strengthens the Immune System | $ 0.00 |
| Encourages Self-Empowerment | $ 0.00 |
| Improves Mood | $ 0.00 |
| Reduces Anxiety & Stress | $ 0.00 |
| Improves Health | $ 0.00 |
| **Total** | **$ 0.00** |

Even after adding in the costs of this book and any massage tools you buy, the benefits of self-massage significantly outweigh its costs. And as Olympic running coach Bobby McGee observes, "the cost-effective aspect of self-massage ensures that the athlete gets work done as regularly as needed."

## Self-Empowering

In the past, athletes heavily depended on medical doctors. That's changing as the burgeoning self-help movement encourages athletes and others to be more responsible for the care of their own bodies. Western medicine's emphasis on cures rather than prevention seems to be eroding as people again become aware that they are ultimately responsible for their own health and that an ounce of prevention is worth a pound of cure. Fortunately, self-massage is as much a preventive therapy as a healing therapy.

That said, still it's common today to hear older athletes say, "I'd rather have someone else give me a massage." This comment may mean, "I'd rather have a massage therapist give me a massage," which is fine. However, when uttered by some men, it seems to mean they're waiting for some model from a Victoria's Secret catalogue to come swooping into their lives and give them a massage. Needless to say, they're likely to be waiting a long time. In any event, self-massage and assisted massage are not mutually exclusive. Athletes can and should have both.

Admittedly, some athletes lack the confidence to effectively practice self-massage. Often this reluctance stems from the mistaken belief they lack a valid standard of comparison. Because massage therapists work on many bodies they can compare one to another. In other words, they can tell you, "Your quads are really tight." Many athletes, especially runners, get a certain satisfaction from hearing a professional tell them how tight their quads are relative to a normal human being. When you act as your own massage therapist, your standard for comparison is you. That can be both an advantage and a disadvantage. It's an advantage because it forces you to compare how you feel at any given moment with how you normally feel or want to feel. It's a disadvantage because it's reassuring to have someone tell you how you feel and how they can make you feel better.

## Immediacy

Because self-massage provides a measure of independence, it can provide an immediate advantage. When you're in the middle of a race you may not have a choice; it's self-massage or DNF*. Dan Brillon, a runner and business executive, was in fourth place at mile-21 of the Leadville Marathon when his right calf suddenly cramped. He says, "It almost brought me down to the ground and was incredibly painful. I was miles away from an aid station so I had no option but to keep moving. I did a combination of self-massage, slow walking for about half a mile, and drinking water with electrolytes to work my way through it. I planned on walking to the next aid station and then dropping out of the race, until a friend pointed out that if I could just jog it into the finish I'd still do pretty well. And that's what I did—managed to hold onto tenth place overall out of 238 finishers. It was an important lesson for me in how to move through a cramp without having it cause an end to my race."

## Getting It When You Need It

Athletes frequently ask: When is the best time to get a massage? Naturally, it's whenever you need one. As triathlete and owner of Skirt Sports Nicole Deboom says, "I use self-massage daily. I really don't have a set schedule. When a specific part of my body needs self-massage, it lets me know. Sometimes it's simply general soreness which is aching for a round of slow gentle flushing. Sometimes I need to dig a little deeper."

---

*Did Not Finish

The best time for you to get a massage may be right before a workout, right after a workout, or even during a workout. Or it may be when you're doing something else, such as watching TV, talking on the telephone, or waiting in traffic. For some athletes the best time for a massage is when they're doing nothing else, when they can devote themselves entirely to their massage. It then becomes a kind of meditation.

For most athletes though, massage is easiest to do while doing something else. Here's how Mike Ricci, triathlete and founder of D3 Multi Sports, put it: "In between workout sessions, almost every night in front of the TV, I work out the knots in my legs or arms from that day's efforts. I usually take the time to figure out what hurts and work around the muscle and then try to just massage out the knots."

If the only time you can find for a massage is when you're doing something else, that's fine. So, when is the best time for you to use self-massage? While

- Watching TV or children
- Reading a book
- Taking a shower
- Thinking about work at the office
- Thinking about work at home
- Relaxing in a hot tub, sauna, or steam room
- Waiting on line
- Riding in planes, trains, and automobiles
- Lying in bed
- Listening to music or watching a movie

## Dual Benefits

One often overlooked advantage of self-massage is its dual nature. While everyone knows the old saying, "It's better to give than to receive," it's clear that with self-massage you do both.

Self-massage pays a twin dividend, giving you two massages for the price of none. Your hands get a massage and the parts of your body they're working get a massage too. Imparting a massage increases your hands' and fingers' flexibility, strength, and range of motion. As seen from your hands' point of view, it's your body that's being used to give your hands a massage.

The very act of massaging carries with it specific benefits. For example, research shows that animal owners get almost as much benefit from petting their pets as their pets do.[1] (Maybe that's why they call them pets.) Additionally, studies demonstrate that elderly people who massage infants show improved mood and self-esteem, and have fewer doctor visits.[2]

## Massaging Your Back

Some athletes won't try self-massage because they can't reach their backs with their hands. They say, "Isn't that what a great massage is all about?" Maybe so but it ignores the fact that you can reach 90 percent of your body with your hands, and you can reach your back with massage tools. Refusing to learn self-massage because you can't reach your back with your hands is like refusing a lifetime supply of free gourmet meals because they don't include asparagus. Yes, it might be nice to have asparagus, but it's not crucial. You can buy asparagus or ask a friend to give you some asparagus.

Furthermore, even the least flexible of us can reach a good portion of our backs with our hands. However, we all can reach our entire back with the right massage tool. The Thera Cane® and Body Back Buddy,™ described in Chapter 16, are particularly effective tools for doing just that.

## Massaging Other People

Few athletes are aware that learning self-massage may be the most effective way to learn to massage a friend or loved one. The way a stroke affects you gives you an idea of how it's likely to affect someone else. Once you're comfortable with the basic massage strokes, you'll be able to apply them confidently to others.

Sometimes just watching self-massage can be a learning experience and get you a free massage to boot. Laurie Edwards, a runner, nursing student and mother, says her six-year-old daughter Aleah learned massage from watching Laurie practice self-massage. Now she gives her mom frequent massages.

## In Summary

All massage has the power to improve the way you feel by relieving sore muscles and helping you recover more quickly between workouts. But only self-massage puts the power directly in your hands. Before moving on to the next chapter, identify the three benefits that you most want to receive from self-massage and write them down.

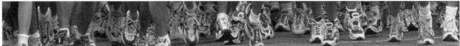

# 3

# Benefits of Massage

## Why Should Anyone Living in the Twenty-First Century Invoke a Medicine That's Older Than Human History?

The best medicine, as the saying goes, is preventive medicine. Preventive medicine is less expensive, easier to administer, and less risky than remedial medicine. As such, massage may be among the best medicines because it is both preventive *and* remedial. If you want to strengthen your immune system and reduce pain, massage is your ticket.

But is massage really medicine? In the United States, we've come to think of medicine as drugs. In the larger picture, though, medicine is much more than that. According to the dictionary, medicine is "the science and art dealing with the maintenance of health and the prevention, alleviation, or cure of disease. . . ."[1] So massage by definition is medicine because it maintains health and prevents and alleviates disease.

While most medicines have short shelf lives, massage has endured. Few medicines last longer than fifty years; fewer still make it a hundred years. Yet massage has been in the race for more than five thousand years and is now experiencing a second wind. In one form or another it's used all over the world. In China it takes the form of *acupressure*; in Japan it's *shiatsu*; in Europe it's *Swedish massage*. You'll find *Tai head massage* in Thailand, *lomi lomi massage* in Hawaii, and the *Turkish bath massage* in Turkey. We in the United States have taken the best from all over the globe, and added some touches of our own.

In the last few hundred years, we've adopted and abandoned scores of medicines including phrenology, lobotomy, and bleeding. Pharmaceuticals that were only a short time ago considered miracle drugs have proven ineffective or harmful. We no longer believe in the efficacy of hundreds of drugs that have been marketed since the 1940s, but we still believe in the power of massage. What is it about massage that makes it so valuable a medicine in so many cultures? Why has it run for thousands of years when so many other therapies have tripped and fallen?

And what about the future of massage? After thousands of years of practice, massage finds itself competing against modern medicine. How will it fare when examined under the microscope of science? Why should anyone in the twenty-first century invoke a medicine that's older than human history? Does it matter that massage healed the pharaohs, that Socrates enjoyed massage, that Jesus employed it, that Buddha found it meditative, and that Freud used it on his patients? How does science say massage is likely to affect your health, fitness, and athletic performance? Those are the questions this chapter seeks to answer.

## Touch

The search for answers to these questions begins with our sense of touch. Touch is not only central to massage, but is our most basic sense. Every living creature experiences the world through touch. It serves as the procreative spark for all creatures and distinguishes pleasure from pain. From an evolutionary perspective, animals that are born without a sense of touch don't survive to reproduce. In fact, all of our other senses are specialized forms of touch. Specialized receptors in our ears sensitive to the touch of sound waves allow us to hear. Our taste buds are specialized receptors sensitive to different-shaped molecules that convey taste. Olfactory-system receptors allow us to touch molecules in the air that produce a sense of smell, while specialized receptors in the eye are sensitized to the touch of light and give us sight.

## Endurance

Massage's power to improve health is the principal reason for its ubiquity from antiquity. As a medicine or healthcare technique, massage predates recorded history. It's likely as old as human life itself, spanning the 150,000 years Homo sapiens have existed.

Massage is part of our natural healthcare system; self-massage is the self-help part of that system. It's as basic to our well-being as bathing, laughing, and loving. It makes us healthy by making us happy, or maybe it's the other way around. No matter how good we think massage is for us, according to the latest science, it's better than that. It's been clinically shown to strengthen the immune system and reduce stress, anxiety, and depression. It makes us feel great. Not even golf can do that!

How do we define massage? One definition is the intentional use of touch to improve health and mood. It can be thought of as an almost instinctive medicine. All humans and mammals massage themselves. Humans use their hands. Less handy mammals use their tongues. Every mother instinctively rubs and massages her baby. We touch and hug those we wish to comfort, and when we're hurt, we instinctively touch and massage our injury. It is this instinct to touch and be touched that is probably at the heart of massage's endurance. Its simplicity may be why we tend to undervalue it. Massage requires little technical knowledge. It's a simple therapy for a complex people.

Massage's simplicity might also explain its endurance. It may be hard to see yourself inventing other therapies, such as surgery, psychoanalysis, or Rolfing, but even if you'd never heard of massage, you could probably imagine yourself inventing self-massage or experimenting with massage on others.

You can imagine a primitive man discovering massage on his own. "Ooo, that feels pretty good," he might say to himself. He might try it on his mate, a friend, or a dog. Before long everyone in the tribe would be rubbing each other. You can see where people might get carried away with it.

"What did you do today, dear?" a wife might ask her husband. "Rubbing, a little bit of rubbing," he might answer. "What else?" she'd ask. "The rubbing took longer than expected," he'd reply. "Weren't you supposed to be hunting?" she'd remind him. You can see where restrictions might have to be implemented to limit rubbing. A professional class might develop whose job it would be to do the rubbing. "Yes, only we can rub," they'd say. "We are the rubbers, I mean doctors." As it turns out, medical doctors practiced massage right up to the middle of the twentieth century.

## Brief History of Massage as Medicine

Twenty-five hundred years ago, the father of Western medicine, Hippocrates, equated medicine with rubbing. Massage was as basic to the healthcare systems of ancient Greece and Rome as drugs are to ours. Of course, massage was around thousands of years before Hippocrates prescribed it for his patients. Every culture that we know of has used massage as a preventive and remedial therapy. It was the primary medicine used throughout the world until pharmaceuticals revolutionized health care in the West just after World War II, replacing massage as the treatment of choice.

Drugs had an immediate powerful effect which proved attractive to patients. Medical doctors were granted a monopoly to prescribe many of these potent new pharmaceuticals. This monopoly gave medical doctors an economic incentive to recommend them over other forms of therapy. Yet in the 1970s, massage became popular again as an integral part of the alternative medicine movement. Since then an increasing body of scientific evidence has been produced to support the rebirth of massage therapy as medicine. This renaissance coincides with a growing disillusionment with drug therapy. Pharmacology schools teach that every drug has two effects: the one we know about and the one we don't. As patients learn more about the harmful effects of drugs, massage, with its thousands of years of history and lack of harmful side effects, has become an attractive alternative.

## The Science of Massage

Until recently, science had little to say about the efficacy of massage. Between the 1940s and 1970s, massage lost its place as an important medical therapy in Western medicine. Medical science devoted its resources to developing new technologies and pharmaceuticals. It wasn't until the 1990s that science began to study the therapeutic value of massage. The result is a growing body of evidence that shows massage to be effective at treating a plethora of healthcare problems.

While this research has been conducted on "massage therapy," that is, one person massaging another, it's likely that similar results would be attained with "self-massage therapy." In fact, all massage, if performed properly, is a form of therapy. Attaching the word "therapy" to "massage" is superfluous. The term "massage therapy" was adopted in the 1970s after the word "massage" had been purloined by the flesh trade as a euphemism for sex.

One reason that so few scientific studies have been conducted on massage, until recently, is money. Scientific studies are expensive. With massage, no large drug companies are willing to pick up the tab because there are no large profits to be made. Indeed, it is estimated to cost between $200 and $500 million to bring the average drug to market.[2] Drugs, over time, can make billions of dollars for the companies that own the exclusive rights to sell them. Not so for massage because no one owns exclusive rights to sell massage. Anyone can do it.

Nevertheless, there has been a recent spate of new studies conducted that show the medical benefits of massage. Beginning in 1992, an impressive body of scientific research on massage began to emerge from the University of Miami School of Medicine. The research funded by Johnson & Johnson, Gerber, and Colgate-Palmolive has been conducted by the Touch Research Institute, headed by Dr. Tiffany Field. It is considered to be the first consistently systematic research done on massage.[3] The results so far suggest that our ancestors got it right by thinking of health care as the art of rubbing.

Scientific research has shown massage provides a number of surprising health benefits. It improves the mood and immune systems of children suffering from cancer,[4] as well as breathing in children suffering from asthma.[5] In studies on women with breast cancer, it has been demonstrated to reduce anxiety and depression and increase immune function.[6] Massage has been shown to relieve chronic fatigue syndrome,[7] post traumatic stress disorder,[8] and hyperactivity associated with Attention Deficit Hyperactivity Disorder.[9] Massage can also enhance alertness and increase job performance.[10] These research findings not only show that massage can effectively treat specific illnesses but that massage is likely to improve health in general. This is good news for athletes whose optimal health is critical for top athletic performance.

In general, research shows that massage produces the following benefits:

- Reduced stress[11]
- Relief from the harmful effects of stress
- Reduced anxiety[12]
- Feeling of well-being
- Fewer illnesses
- Elevated mood
- Relief from pain[13]
- Feelings of pleasure
- Improved sleep[14]
- Calm energy
- Reduced depression[15]
- Relaxed body and mind
- Relief from premenstrual syndrome (PMS)[16]
- Enhanced alertness[17]
- Relief from migraine headaches[18]
- Relief from asthma[19]
- Increased job performance[20]

- Better understanding of yourself
- Relief from eating disorders[21]
- Increased self-confidence

## Core Benefits of Massage

While science continues to conduct research into the mysteries of massage, it has already identified three **core** benefits of massage. In test after test, and study after study, the results show that

1. Massage improves health;
2. Massage elevates mood;
3. Massage reduces pain.

Massage doesn't just treat injuries and illnesses in the way traditional Western medicine does. It improves health, that is, it improves the function of the entire human being. Traditional Western medicine is relatively effective at dealing with severe illness and injury, but it does little to improve general health. If you're unlucky enough to get hit by a car and suffer multiple internal injuries, Western medicine is the best bet for patching you up. But if you were unhealthy before you were hit, even if your doctors resolved all of the injuries resulting from the car crash, you're still going to be unhealthy when you recover.

Massage works its healthcare magic in two ways. First, it strengthens the immune system.[22] Second, it improves circulation, which can serve to feed and clean every cell in your body. As a result, massage has the potential to improve the function of every living part of you.

## Stress

The most important way massage strengthens our immune system is by reducing stress. Stress is a natural biological response to any disruption caused by a physical, mental, or emotional event. It can be a healthy reaction, typically associated with the "fight-or-flight" response. When you feel threatened, your body responds to the perceived danger by releasing a flood of hormones into your bloodstream, including cortisol and adrenaline. Blood pressure and heart rate increase, and the digestive processes are interrupted to deal with the perceived danger. These changes serve to focus attention, increase strength, extend endurance, and improve reaction time. These responses have survival value if you're under physical attack. If not, they are at best wasteful, and at worst destructive.

Excess stress is a serious problem for most people. It is estimated that seventy-five percent of all visits to primary care physicians are related to stress. Excess stress can be especially significant for athletes who continually push their bodies to compete.

Because much of modern stress is a response to psychological rather than physical threats, for many of us these perceived threats never cease. Our bodies continually react as if we are under attack, fighting a fight that doesn't exist while creating health problems that do. Excessive stress makes us more susceptible to illness of all kinds. It affects our mood and bodily functions including sleep patterns and eating behavior.

At the heart of the problem is the release of a group of hormones, including cortisol, into the blood. These hormones reduce the function of the immune system. Cortisol also correlates with increased appetite and weight gain. It appears to act as a sedative which can cause depression, and has been shown to cause loss of sex drive, which in itself is depressing. Elevated levels of cortisol correlate with raised heart rate and increased blood pressure, cholesterol and triglyceride levels, all of which increase the risk of heart attack and stroke. High cortisol levels also increase abdominal fat which correlates with increased risk of diabetes. All of these risk factors are acceptable if experienced infrequently when a fight-or-flight response is appropriate. However, when experienced continually, high cortisol levels are dangerous.[23] Fortunately, according to clinical tests, massage reduces levels of cortisol in the blood and reduces stress.[24]

## Circulation

There is something almost magical in the touching of skin by skin. Physically, it increases the flow of blood and improves circulation. It gives the human being a calm, relaxed energy. Only massage conveys this feeling, and nothing else compares to it. Both science and experience tell us that massage stirs the blood, warms the skin, and relaxes the body. We may not need science to tell us that stroking our bare skin with a warm hand will warm our skin and increase circulation. We may not need science to tell us that massage relaxes the body and the mind; that it relieves tension and reduces stress.[25] But it's nice to discover that scientific research verifies our experiences.

Research shows that massage has a local and systemic effect

on blood flow.[26] Increased circulation accelerates the flow of oxygen and nutrients to our cells and the cleansing of waste products from our cells. Massage allows us to target increased circulation to those areas of our body that need it most.

## Pain

Massage has been shown to be an effective analgesic. Clinical research shows that massage relieves pain in many of the ways that humans suffer from it, including labor pains and pain from PMS, migraine headaches, juvenile rheumatoid arthritis, and fibromyalgia.[27] Science is uncertain just how massage reduces pain so ubiquitously. It has been speculated that certain forms of massage may produce endorphin cocktails, and these chemical substances mediate pain. Additional research needs to be done in this area.

## Mood

Scientific research has shown that massage improves mood. If you've ever had a relaxing massage you know massage lifts your spirits.

Clinical tests have shown massage reduces anxiety—a state of unease, fear, or worry—in children, adolescents,[28] and women during childbirth.[29] It's likely to do the same for athletes but there have been no clinical trials to substantiate this hypothesis. You might test this theory on your own. The next time you're anxious about a competition or an event, get a massage and see if your anxiety is reduced.

Massage can reduce depression in adolescent mothers[30] and improve the behavior and health of infants of depressed mothers.[31] It's also been shown to reduce depression (along with stress and anxiety) in those suffering from chronic fatigue syndrome.[32]

By reducing stress, anxiety, depression, and pain, massage improves mood. Reducing all four will inexorably improve health. Regular massage elevates mood in ways pharmaceutical executives can only dream about. Massage may be more effective at improving mood than Prozac,[33] Zoloft, and other psychopharmaceuticals. Although no clinical trials have thus far been conducted to validate this hypothesis, one issue is settled: massage, unlike pharmaceuticals, has no harmful side effects. All its side effects are healthful. When done properly, it can unite mind, body, and spirit, and give you a buzz that lasts all day. Again no clinical tests have been performed, but you can substantiate this finding on your own.

# The Limits of Science

Thirty-five years ago there were about ten licensed massage schools in the U.S.; today there are 1,200. It is estimated that Americans spend from $4 to $6 billion on massage annually and make more than 100 million visits to massage therapy offices.[34] These numbers not only reflect the public's growing awareness of the importance of massage, but a need for more research into the medical effects of massage. Because modern medicine relies on scientific testing as authority for efficacy, testing is one useful way to evaluate massage and compare its effectiveness to other treatments. Until recently, science has neglected massage, but that is changing as Americans rediscover the benefits of massage.

It is hoped that science will continue to study massage and expand the scope and depth of its research to include studies to show how massage and self-massage affect health in the general population, as well as studies on sports massage. As of this writing, science has barely scratched the surface on what is arguably one of the most accessible cost-effective medicines available.

Unfortunately, science is unlikely to expand its scope in the near future. The chief problem is funding. Because quality research is costly, unless a corporation or university is likely to financially gain from the research, it is unlikely to be conducted.

The good news is that while scientific research is important for massage, it is not critical for its survival. Many of the benefits of massage need not be verified by science because they can be verified by the end user, you. In fact, it is simpler and more effective in most cases for you to verify the benefits of massage than for you to rely on science. It's easy to do by either going to a massage therapist, enlisting a friend, or practicing self-massage. This way you can discover what does and doesn't work for you.

You may not need science to validate how massage affects you any more than you need a weatherman to tell you which way the wind is blowing. Medical research, in general, evaluates the effect of a medicine on the general population, in short, the average person. It conducts research using a large-enough sample to make reliable inferences about the population at large and to discover how the average person will respond. The scientific approach is crucial in research involving acute medical conditions such as cancer, cardiovascular disease, or Alzheimer's disease. The medical technologies needed to treat these illnesses are extremely expensive to develop. Scientific evidence is the best way to evaluate their efficacy and direct scarce resources to where they will do the most good.

The drugs and technologies used to treat these conditions are often dangerous and sometimes deadly. As Dr. Andrew Weil has observed, "the only difference between a drug and a poison is dose. All drugs become poisons in high enough doses and many poisons become useful drugs in low enough doses."[35] It makes economic sense to use scientific methods to evaluate these potentially lethal treatments because we cannot safely test them ourselves. It's not as important to use scientific methods with massage because we can each safely test massage for ourselves.

Even if there were an abundance of scientific research available on massage it would make sense for you to do your own research. Medical science tells us how the average person benefits from massage, not how you will benefit. Your inner-biology is as unique to you as is your face. The best way to find out how you will benefit from massage is to discover it for yourself.

## Benefits of Frequent Massage

Whether you rely on science or your own experience, you will probably find that frequent massage is the best massage. According to studies from the University of Miami at the Touch Research Institute (TRI), if you want to enjoy the most important health benefits of massage, regular massage is important. Getting a massage once a month or even once a week is probably not enough to strengthen your immune system. Most research on adults done by the TRI involve two thirty-minute sessions per week. It is likely that more frequent massage would be even more effective. The studies at TRI were limited to two sessions per week for what were termed "practical considerations, namely that most adults could not afford more than two half-hour sessions per week by a professional or by a significant other."[36] Self-massage removes these limitations.

Research shows that massage reduces stress, anxiety, and depression in subjects receiving massage no fewer than twice per week.[37] These reductions likely elevate the immune system and improve health. So, if you want to enjoy improved health, you should have no fewer than two massages per week, according to the best science available on the subject. These results, of course, reflect what the average person is likely to experience. If you want to know how best to improve your health, conduct your own research, either by hiring a massage therapist, engaging a significant other, or using self-massage.

When beginning your massage program, use scientific research as a guide. If you wish to improve your health, start with two thirty-minute massages per week. After four weeks, evaluate your results, and make adjustments as necessary. If you want to reduce muscle pain and soreness, try a massage as soon as you experience soreness. If you want to reduce your recovery time, try a massage after every workout. And if you want to feel better all the time, try a daily massage. Through experimentation, you'll find what works best for you.

No one knows just how beneficial regular massage may be for you. Frequent massage may improve your health as much as quitting smoking improves a smoker's health. Daily massage may be as advantageous as a healthy diet or a regular workout. The best way to find out is to experiment on your own.

## In Summary

When practiced regularly, massage will significantly improve your health and mood. With improved health, you'll be able to train more consistently, improving your fitness and athletic performance.

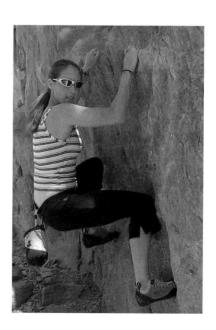

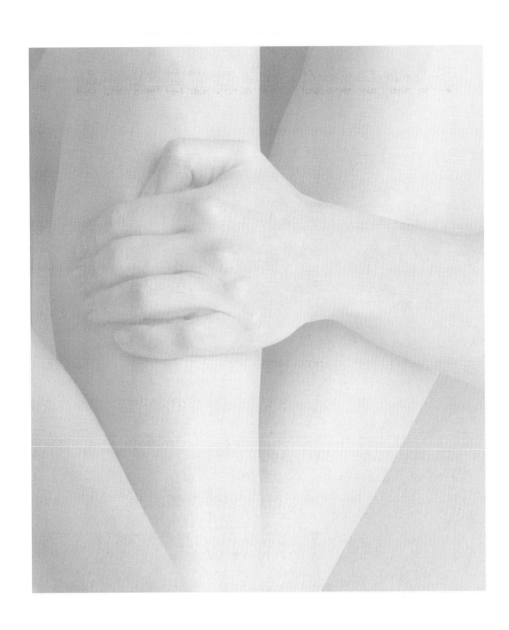

# 4

# Why Your Body Needs Massage

How Massage Affects Every Living Part of You

## The Science of Touching

Because we cannot be touched without being changed, touch changes our world, both internally and externally. From a systems perspective, touch is an information system, relaying information about pain, temperature, pressure, and pleasure. It is also an energy transfer system, through which mechanical energy is transferred to our skin as heat energy and through our skin as biochemical and electrical energy. Biochemical energy travels through our blood as part of our blood chemistry. Electrical energy travels through our nervous system to our brain where it informs us of possibilities.

Touch is our most direct way of receiving information about our immediate environment and of satisfying a multitude of physical needs. Massage, a form of intentional touch, is the art and science of meeting those needs. As discussed in the prior chapter, massage is part of a natural healthcare system that reduces pain, produces pleasure, increases our immune system's function, warms our skin and muscles, increases circulation, helps us heal, and improves our overall health. Massage accomplishes these tasks through a network of energy and information transfer.

As you rub your hand along the surface of your arm during a massage, *boom*, you convert mechanical energy to heat energy on both the skin surface of your arm and your hand. Below your skin, the mechanical energy and heat energy produce electrical and chemical energy. Chemicals in the form of endorphins, hormones, and enzymes are released into your blood stream. Nerves carry information in the form of electrical energy which is transmitted between nerves by chemical substances called neurotransmitters. In this way, information is transmitted all over your body. Word gets out, "Free Massage Tonight." Different parts of your body volunteer; "me next, me next," they say. Your body communicates its needs to your hands, and your hands answer those needs. Your body knows what will make it feel best and your hands do the rest.

## Your Magic Skin

Because massage begins with skin, it's good to know a little bit about your outer limits. So here's the skinny on skin. Skin is your largest, oldest, and most sensitive sense organ. It weighs about nine pounds and covers about 18 square feet in area. The shape of your skin is the shape you're in. It fits, well, like a skin. No matter how much pasta you eat, you never outgrow your skin. Sometimes it looks a lot better in clothes.

Your skin is both simple and complex. Like Silly-Putty, it's flexible and bounces a little. You can even write on it. Your skin keeps your insides inside you. It's waterproof on the outside but leaks from the inside. It protects you from the thousand natural shocks that flesh is heir to, including physical injury, dehydration, overheating, and ultraviolet light. In addition to being beautiful to look at and pleasurable to touch, your skin is a warning system. It alerts you that something hard, soft, cold, wet, sharp, pointed, or dangerous is touching you. As athletes, we know skin helps regulate our body's temperature, hydration, and electrolyte levels through sweat. A section of skin the size of a quarter contains three feet of blood vessels, fifty nerve endings, thousands of sweat glands, and a few million cells.[1] Because of all the wonderful things it does, it may be best to think of your skin as magic.

While skin under a microscope is complex stuff, skin to the touch is simple enough. Touching it can arouse you or relax you. In fact, to keep your skin working properly, it's necessary to touch it.

## Your Information Network

Your outer layer of skin, the epidermis, is where you begin. Under the epidermis is the dermis. Touching your dermis from the inside are millions of nerve endings whose job is to communicate with every other cell in your body. Your nerve cells tell you what's happening outside you—what's hot and what's not, what's there and what's air. When something touches you, the sensation passes through your skin to your nerve cells, which spread the news, in the form of electricity, all over your body. These electrical sensations form an intelligence that tells you how you feel so that you can help yourself feel better. It's important to learn to listen to these sensations.

## Your Blood

You are billions of cells. It's their life that makes up your life. Blood keeps every one of them alive and alert by transferring energy and information to them. By affecting the flow of blood, massage affects the flow of information and energy throughout your body.

At the cellular level, your blood serves as a combination room-service, maid-service, and wake-up service. It feeds your cells, it cleans them, and it informs them. Blood feeds and informs your cells by delivering oxygen, nutrients, chemicals, endorphins, enzymes, and hormones. Blood cleans them by carting away the messy waste produced from cellular meals. If your cells are not fed, cleaned, and informed, they perform poorly. By increasing the flow of blood, massage helps boost your cells' performance.

According to Dr. Andrew Weil, "A healthy circulatory system with healthy and normal blood, is the keystone of the body's healing system. One of the most effective ways to promote healing, if it can be done, is to increase the amount of blood reaching an ailing part of the body."[2] After a hard workout, your blood is loaded with waste produced by your muscles. Gradually your blood carries these waste products away. By increasing the flow of oxygen-rich blood to your muscles, massage speeds up the cleaning process, feeding your muscles and helping them rebuild more quickly.

In addition to increasing circulation, massage strokes affect blood chemistry. Massage stirs your natural chemistry and re-leases healthful biochemicals—an endorphin cocktail, stirred but not shaken—including enzymes, peptides, hormones, dopamine, anandamide, and of course, endorphins. As mentioned in Chapter 3, massage speeds the removal of cortisol from your blood, a chemical that causes stress and has been shown to suppress the immune system.[3]

After a workout, your blood is as tired as you are. Most athletes don't have a feel for the shape their blood is in after hard exercise, and science doesn't have a handy test you can perform on yourself to assess the health of your blood after a workout. However, there is one person who is an expert on blood, and he would be happy to test it for you.

# The Dracula Test

The truth is that modern science does not fully understand blood. It thinks it does with its fancy words like hemoglobin and corpuscles. But medical doctors don't really get blood. The only one who really gets blood is Dracula. "I drink it because it tastes good," he says. "And it's so good for you." Dracula's favorite blood is fresh blood from healthy athletic specimens. He likes clean, healthy, oxygenated blood, or at least that's how he's portrayed in old movies. Dracula certainly would not touch your blood after a workout. He'd shiver just to think how dirty, smelly, and polluted it is.

If it's not good enough for Dracula, it shouldn't be good enough for you. Massage cleans it up, refreshes it, feeds it, and rejuvenates it. Here's the question you should ask yourself after a workout: Would Dracula gag on my blood? If the answer is yes, you need a massage!

# Modern Medicine

All of us who are alive in the twenty-first century owe a debt of gratitude to modern medical science and the many health benefits it has brought us. But let's not lose sight of the fact that sooner or later almost every new scientific "fact" relating to modern medicine will be proven wrong or be in need of substantial revision. Two hundred years from now, people will look back at our modern medicine with the same sense of wonder that we look back at the way Western medicine was practiced two hundred years ago.

Since every athlete is a unique biological experiment, the medical discoveries that you should embrace are those that you make about yourself. In other words, it's up to you, not science, to discover how you work. If you wait for science to discover what's going on inside you, you're in for a long wait or worse. Because science does not generally explore the healthy among us, if your health is fragile enough to be investigated by medical science, you're likely to be in mortal danger. So if medical science has not set its sights on exploring you, that's good. If you're exploring yourself, that's also good, because that's how you'll find out about yourself. What matters ultimately is what people feel.

## The Genie Hypothesis

Medical science cannot fully account for all the good things massage produces inside the human body. Some athletes like to think there's a genie inside them that produces many of these benefits. Medical doctors argue against the existence of internal genies but as some athletes have discovered, experience and imagination may be better teachers than science. Many athletes like the genie metaphor because it presents a visual image of what they feel happening inside them. When they rub the magic lamp that is their body, they awaken the genie, an energy, and a force in themselves that makes them feel great.

## In Summary

Self-massage is a way of transferring energy and information to cleanse and feed every cell in your body. Massage produces its powerful effects by converting mechanical energy to thermal, electrical, and chemical energy. When performing self-massage, visualize this energy and cleansing system working. If you don't want to remember the electrochemical energy transfer stuff, do what many athletes do. Visualize a genie inside you whose powers are awakened by massage. What matters ultimately is what you feel.

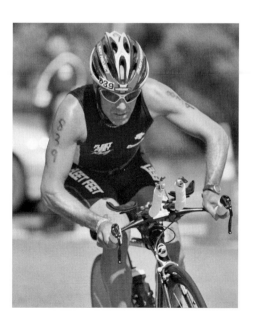

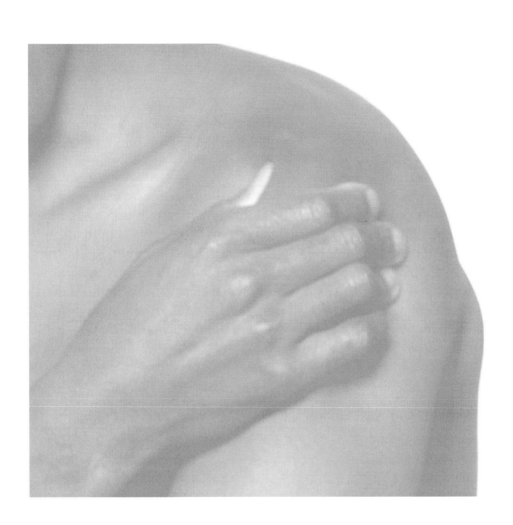

# 5

# Sports Massage

## Improving Your Athletic Performance with Massage

*"I started getting sports massages and realized what a wonderful thing it is for your body."*— Martina Navratilova

In addition to being a wonderful thing for your body, sports massage gives you a competitive edge. It improves fitness and athletic performance by allowing you to train more effectively, that is, more often, with less pain.

No matter what sport you play, massage will improve your performance. Whether you measure that improvement in terms of strength, speed, fitness, or pleasure is up to you. That's what makes learning self-massage a smart investment of your time and effort.

## What Is Sports Massage?

Sports massage is massage used to improve athletic performance. It's been used for that purpose for more than twenty-five hundred years—from the first Olympic Games of ancient Greece to the games of the twenty-first century.

Sports massage can help you prepare for, perform during, or recover between workouts.[1] Incorporating sports massage into your training program will improve your athletic performance by preventing injuries, and by improving health and mood. For many athletes, improved performance means increased pleasure, but sports massage increases your pleasure in more direct ways. It releases endorphin cocktails, reduces muscle pain, and boosts self-confidence. If sports massage were a drug, it might be banned for giving competitors too great an advantage.

Athletes know their bodies can give them enormous pleasure as well as enormous pain. Sports massage is a simple way to create balance between the pain and pleasure produced by exercise. Many athletes, it seems, are more comfortable with pain than pleasure. If the pleasure of massage makes you feel guilty, think of massage as a way of restoring balance to your body. Lance Armstrong said he didn't ride for pleasure, and described pain as transcendent.[2] Even so, Lance took advantage of massage whenever he could.[3]

In addition to giving you pleasure, sports massage will give you many other benefits. According to professional athletes, massage therapists, and physicians, sports massage

- Prepares muscles for workouts
- Increases range of motion
- Reduces risk of injury
- Reduces muscle pain and soreness
- Reduces muscle tension
- Releases endorphin cocktails
- Speeds recovery between workouts
- Stimulates and relaxes
- Improves muscle tone and flexibility
- Improves health and mood

Sports massage can unleash these powerful benefits with little effort and expense. With sports massage, you can make yourself feel better than the average athlete, any time you want.

## Professional Athletes Do It

Professional athletes did it and still do it. Babe Ruth, Muhammad Ali, Chris Evert, Michael Jordan, and Joe Montana did it. Lance Armstrong did it and does it. Sally Edwards, Peggy Fleming, Steve Prefontaine, and Arnold Palmer did it. Tiger Woods and Frank Shorter do it. Martina Navratilova did it, does it, and is still talking about it. Mark Allen and Dave Scott did it in Hawaii. Mickey Mantle, Jean-Claude Killy, and Pelé did it. Mia Hamm still does it and always will do it. All are past, present, or future users of sports massage. They use it to prepare for and recover from workouts. The list of every professional athlete who has used massage to enhance their athletic performance would fill a book the size of the Manhattan telephone directory.

The great, the near-great, and the not-so-great of professional sport use massage for the same reasons you should. Lilly Guerra Johnson past winner of the Bolder Boulder, and one of the more engaging athletes in Boulder, Colorado, put it this way: "Massage is important when you want to perform at your best."

Professional athletes use massage to help recover from workouts because quick recovery is essential for all athletes. Mark Allen, six-time winner of the Hawaiian Ironman Triathlon, believes that massage was an indispensable part of his training: just as athletes need hard work to excel, they also need massage to quicken recovery between workouts, prevent injuries, and reduce stress.[4]

World class athletes often credit massage with keeping them healthy and preventing injury. Elite triathlete Marco Coelho agrees: "Massage helps me avoid injury. It reduces my muscle tension and stress. Bodywork, especially, massage should be part of every athlete's training."

Elite runner Laurie Edwards described the benefits of massage this way: "After I started getting regular massages, I could see how much they helped my running." She learned self-massage from paying attention when getting professional sports massage and now she uses self-massage every day. She says, "without massage and self-massage, I don't believe I would be able to run today at all."

Almost every professional sports team that can afford one has a professional massage therapist on staff. Almost every professional athlete who can afford one uses a professional massage therapist. If you only received the benefits those athletes do, sports massage would give you a huge advantage. But with self-massage you may enjoy many more benefits than professional athletes.

## Doing It Before, During, and After Workouts

Every athlete has a favorite time to practice sports massage. For most, it's related directly to their workouts because massage is a great way to warm up your body. It also comes in handy during a workout if a muscle tenses up. And finally, right after a workout, massage is a great way to relax, relieve muscle soreness, and speed recovery. Not surprisingly, it's convenient to divide sports massage into three phases: (1) pre-workout massage, (2) workout massage, and (3) post-workout massage.

## Pre-Workout Massage

The pre-workout massage literally warms you up. It's a short five-to-ten-minute massage that rouses your body and relaxes your mind. It uses light, stimulating, drumming strokes and gliding strokes of light to moderate pressure. The light gliding strokes warm your skin while moderate pressure and light drumming strokes increase your circulation and heart rate.

By heating and activating your muscles, your pre-workout massage prepares you for the stress that's about to come. Working directly on a muscle decreases muscle tension by expanding and warming it, thus reducing your risk of injury and increasing your range of motion.

The pre-workout massage also focuses your attention where it should be before a workout: on your body. It begins the process of connecting your conscious thoughts with your body. This centering of attention reduces stress and anxiety while increasing self-confidence. For many athletes massage is more effective than stretching because you're less likely to tear a cold, stiff muscle warming it up with massage than warming it up with stretching.[5]

Physically stimulating and psychologically sedating, massage simultaneously arouses and relaxes you. It works in the same way that walking or light exercise works to produce a calm, almost relaxed, energy. This calm energy is a particularly good way to begin your workout or competition.

## Workout Massage

The purpose of massage during your workout or competition is to address an immediate problem and to prevent a minor problem from growing into a major one. Massage can help you complete a competition when a muscle cramps up. In the midst of a long run or climb, it is a way to relax and ease tension. It can be performed between innings in a baseball game or before eating one of your young during a rugby match. Cyclists often massage their neck, shoulders, or quads during long rides. Most minor muscle problems can be resolved quickly and effectively with a few strokes and pokes, leaving you feeling better.

Professional triathlete Nicole Deboom says,

> I have always been a bit of a cramper. I'm talking about cramps that start in the hamstrings and make their way around to the front of your legs and down into your calves. During my first

Ironman, 2000 Ironman California, I was leading the race for much of the day. I knew the hamstring cramps were starting to form; I was essentially waiting to see how they would affect me. As I was being passed, the hamstrings started to flare up. I still had 6 miles to go; I needed to hold strong and keep those leg cramps at bay. I was forced into a walk, but that wasn't enough. I found the spot at the attachment of the muscle and applied some pressure. I could feel the muscle relax and release. It was just enough to start running again. I used the same method three or four more times; all I needed at that point was to make it to the finish. Without the innate knowledge of my body's needs that self-massage nurtures, I may not have known how to alleviate those cramps. I was able to cross the line in third place at my first-ever Ironman, inciting a five-year Ironman career that culminated in a win at Ironman Wisconsin in 2004.

## Post-Workout Massage

The post-workout massage helps you recover from your workout. It's a more intense, longer massage, lasting twenty to sixty minutes. The post-workout massage doesn't have to be done directly after your workout to be effective. You can perform it the next day and still receive most, if not all, of its benefits. Among its rewards, a good post-workout massage:

- Reduces muscle pain and tension
- Relieves delayed onset muscle soreness (DOMS)[6]
- Restores and increases range of motion[7]
- Restores and improves muscle tone and flexibility
- Restores and improves fitness by speeding recovery
- Heals soft tissue injury
- Releases endorphin cocktails
- Prevents injury

Its first effect is warming. Warm skin increases circulation which provides fresh nutrients and oxygen-rich blood. Blood heals, fuels, and flushes toxins from your cells. This warming process soothes and relieves tension in your sore muscles. In addition, by lengthening your sore muscles, massage restores and improves your flexibility and range of motion. The post-workout massage helps you identify and treat small injuries before they become large injuries.

Massage also reduces the likelihood that you will be sore the day after a tough workout. It has been shown that massage helps athletes recuperate from fatigue more effectively than rest alone.[8] More intense massage strokes release endorphin cocktails that reduce pain, produce pleasure, and create a sense of well-being.

## Injury Prevention

All three types of massage invite you to explore your body by:

- Directing your attention to strengths and weaknesses
- Caring for areas of soreness and tightness

By focusing your attention on those places where you're most vulnerable to injury and making you aware of your weaknesses, massage reduces the likelihood that you will overtrain, that is, work out on days you really should rest. That's one reason massage is effective at preventing sports-related injuries.

Sports massage helps prevent injuries in three other ways. First, it helps you recover more fully from your last workout, making you stronger and less likely to be injured during your next workout. Second, massage improves flexibility, which reduces the likelihood that you'll suffer torn, strained, or pulled muscles. As you learn to identify tight muscles, you can use self-massage to reduce their tension. You may notice that as your muscles become more flexible, your movements become more fluid. And fluidity, as everyone knows, is the mark of a great athlete.

The third, and most important, way that massage reduces injuries is to catch them while they're small. As the philosopher Lao Tzu observed 3,000 years ago, "the biggest problem in the world could have been solved when it was small." Most sports injuries start as small imperceptible weaknesses and grow into large overuse injuries. Massage helps repair them before they have a chance to interfere with your training. As Dr. Weil observes, "The earlier you notice a medical problem, the less work will be needed to correct it. . . . The farther into its course a disease proceeds before therapeutic measures are applied, the stronger the measures need to be and the smaller their chance of succeeding."[9]

## Recovery

Because working out is an injury to your muscles, every time you work out you get weaker, not stronger. It's during the period *following* your workout that your muscles recover, heal, and grow stronger. That's why recovery is crucial. To get fitter faster, learn to recover faster. Massage speeds recovery after your last workout so that you're ready to benefit more fully from your next workout. With full recovery, your training becomes more effective and more enjoyable, making you better able to reach your training goals.

To better understand training, it's helpful to divide it into two phases: the workout phase and the recovery phase. They go together like night and day, like sleeping and waking. If you don't sleep, you don't perform well. If you don't recover, your muscles don't perform well.

The workout phase is that part of your training that wears your muscles down. The recovery phase is the training that allows your muscles to adapt, heal, and grow stronger. Both are essential. If you haven't recovered after a workout, you're wasting your time working out again.

Lack of recovery can lead to overtraining. The first symptom you'll notice is sore muscles or joints. As time goes by, and you fail to recover, you'll feel continual aches and pains. You may have trouble sleeping. Your muscles will feel tense, and your mind anxious. If you ignore these symptoms you're likely to suffer more of them. Your performance will decline and even the pleasure you may have gotten from pain will disappear.

To avoid injury, athletes need to allow themselves to recover. When overtraining, all athletes become susceptible to injuries such as strains, sprains, breaks, falls, crashes, and collapses. Injuries like these are generally not accidents; they happen because of incomplete recovery.

According to Neal Henderson, MS, CSCS, coordinator of sports medicine for the Boulder Center for Sports Medicine:

> Many athletes are under mistaken impressions with regard to training that they need to force their body into severe discomfort consistently to improve. While there are times for this type of effort in training, consistently doing this is not helpful. By paying attention to your own body, and learning how different muscle groups are responding to varied efforts, they can begin to truly know how their body is responding over time by using self-massage.

## A Coach's Recovery Story

Most athletes doubt they need to recover after working out. Young athletes especially tend to believe the best way to get stronger is to work out more intensely and more often. Coach Wu, a legendary California running coach, explained the importance of recovery to his high school runners this way:

One day after a hard workout, Coach Wu gathered his whole team together in the gym. He patiently explained the importance of recovery. He was a thoughtful coach and spoke softly. At the end of his talk, he said, "Anyone who doesn't understand the importance of recovery raise your hand. Now, the ten of you who raised your hands, I want you to get up and run into that wall."

Five of the ten runners immediately understood the need for recovery. The other five stood up and ran into the wall. They hit it hard, and some looked a little dazed lying on the floor. The coach looked at them with concern. With compassion in his voice, he said, "Any of you who still don't understand the meaning of recovery get up and do it again. Until you understand the meaning of recovery, you're going to keep running into that wall."

Sports massage is a way of speeding your recovery, allowing you to work out more effectively and more often, and avoid hitting that wall.

## Endorphin Cocktails

When performed effectively, sports massage releases endorphin cocktails into your system to reduce pain. One of the skills you're training when working out is your ability to effectively respond to pain. Your body responds to pain by releasing its natural pain-killers—endorphin cocktails. Massage also releases these natural analgesics, which not only reduce pain but make you feel good.

## In Summary

Don't worry if you've never performed a sports massage. You'll learn how in Part II of this book. Right now all you need is an understanding of how massage can help you achieve your athletic goals, prevent injuries, and speed recovery.

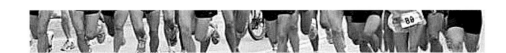

# 6

# Endorphins

### Activating Your Endorphin
### Delivery System with Self-Massage

*"The sage is guided by what he feels and not by what he sees."*—Lao Tzu

Strong scientific evidence suggests that all animals have a system for reducing pain and producing pleasure. For human beings that system can be activated through self-massage. It involves, at least in part, endorphins. It also involves a shaker full of other biochemicals produced by your body which affect pain and pleasure. They include adrenaline, serotonin ("the molecule of happiness)[1], dopamine ("the molecule of desire")[2], and anandamide[3] ("the bliss receptor").[4] These and other biochemicals working to mediate pain and pleasure are collectively called endorphin cocktails[5]. This chapter focuses on the endorphin component of the mix because it is the biochemical most closely associated with athletes. Much research has been conducted on endorphins, although much more needs to be done relating to athletes.

In the 1970s, science discovered what the human body had known for tens of thousands of years: when physically stressed, the human body produces chemicals to reduce that stress.[6] These chemicals are called endorphins. As athletes, we have probably developed a better endorphin delivery system than non-athletes. That's because workouts train our endorphin system to deliver; that is, to reduce pain and produce pleasure.

Think of endorphins as the superheroes of our nervous system. They come to our rescue to block pain when we stress our bodies during long runs and intense physical exertion. But unlike Batman, endorphins don't always respond to our call.

Sometimes they show up and we feel great and perform at our best. Other times they don't show up and we feel weak and perform poorly. No one knows why.

# Endorphins Defined

Endorphins are analgesic euphorics. Chains of amino acids called peptides, they reduce pain, produce pleasure, and serve as powerful evolutionary forces. Chemically, endorphins resemble opiates, such as morphine. All mammals produce them. They've been shaping behavior in human beings and our mammalian ancestors for millions of years, so it is startling that they weren't discovered by science until 1975.

In 1973, scientists found specialized receptors in the brain that accept morphine. They theorized that the brain must produce its own morphine-like substance to fit into these receptors. Two years later, three groups of scientists, working independently, found this to be the case. They called these substances, "endorphins," short for endogenous morphine, or "morphine created internally." Like morphine, endorphins relieve pain and produce pleasure.

# Morphine vs. Endorphins

Although chemically similar to morphine, endorphins are not exactly the same. Some types of endorphins were found to be one hundred times more powerful than morphine.[7] Overall, endorphins are more fun, effective, powerful, and for athletes, much more useful. Consider these differences: morphine is produced in a lab from a flower, the opium poppy. Endorphins are produced by the human body for the human body. Morphine was invented in 1803 by a German druggist. Endorphins evolved first in mammals and then in humans over millions of years. Morphine is a foreign substance shown to have harmful side effects. Endorphins are a natural product of the human body with no known harmful side effects. Morphine makes us see things that are not there. Endorphins make us see things that are there more clearly. No one is going to rob you to satisfy their endorphin habit. Endorphins are free, legal, and they make you feel better.

Endorphins are neither ingested nor injected. They are produced by your body when needed and in the quantities needed. As an athlete, you produce them when your muscles are stressed by exercise intensity or duration. Even so, you may need a little help producing them, and that's where self-massage can prove valuable.

# Healthcare System

Massage is basically an instinctive healthcare modality or medicine. We hold and caress those we wish to comfort. When we hurt ourselves, our first reaction is to touch and rub the hurt. A universal maternal behavior, massage is part of all cultures' traditional healthcare systems. The production of endorphins is probably at the heart of this system. We know that both endorphins and massage reduce pain and produce pleasure. Scientists have theorized that endorphins released during massage are the underlying cause of the pleasure you feel.

From an evolutionary perspective, it's easy to see how our early ancestors would have been attracted to massage. Because they had little except their hands and their bodies, it's easy to imagine that, huddled in caves, they discovered that by running their hands over their bodies and applying pressure to their muscles they felt better, healthier, happier. It was one of our first healthcare systems.

Imagine the benefits of a healthcare system based on touch, wired into our very beings. Self-massage encouraged early humans to explore and learn about their bodies. Because it is a healing system based on touch, it brought people together, promoting affection, bonding, and intimacy. Such a system would have been a strong component of any early pre-tribal culture because it would encourage social dependence and intimate relationships between people. This in turn would have helped them form social units in which to raise children. It's easy to see how massage had survival value and why natural selection would favor those of our early ancestors who used it.

A healthcare system based on touch also encouraged our ancestors to explore the world with their hands in the same way they explored their bodies. It led them to use their hands to manipulate their environment, to touch, to heal, to fix, to create.

In Asia, this ancient system of health care evolved into a system of acupressure and acupuncture; it is at the heart of traditional Chinese medicine. While modern Western medicine may have abandoned massage, many Westerners have not.

# Endorphin Continuum

Massage is instinctively used as a first means of self treatment. When you hurt yourself, your immediate reaction is to touch and rub the painful part. Similarly, you caress those you wish to comfort when they are hurt. It is likely that one effect of such touching is the release of small amounts of endorphins.

Your body also produces endorphins in response to physical stress. The quantities you produce vary along a continuum. The more physical stress your body is under, the more endorphins you're likely to produce. In life-threatening situations, you produce huge quantities of endorphins along with adrenaline and other neurotransmitters. These substances help you think more clearly and act more swiftly to avoid injury and death. Time itself appears to slow down to give you time to act and save yourself.

Life-threatening events and extreme sports both provoke peak endorphin experiences. Two distinct types of peak endorphin experiences relate to sports. The first takes place during the athletic event, the second after the athletic event. Occurring rarely, both eliminate pain, produce a sense of euphoria, and involve altered states of consciousness. Although they're infrequent, most athletes have experienced them at one time or another.

An endorphin peak during an athletic event is a mysterious but welcome experience. As your bloodstream fills with endorphins, you begin to sense things differently. Everything becomes clear as your mind and body fuse with your activity. You feel calm and powerful, almost invincible. Your body is no longer a limiting factor. It's almost as if it has fallen away. As physical pain disappears, your attention is effortlessly focused in the moment, in your motion, and on your intention. At times you almost feel like you're watching yourself. Again, time seems to slow. Objects become more vivid. Targets may expand in size.

Such an intense endorphin experience is probably a survival tool. The same feeling people report in near-death experiences, it's likely that the endorphin peak is programmed to occur as a defense against death. Because it usually occurs when physical and emotional stress is extreme,[8] this kind of endorphin peak is sometimes triggered during athletic events, as almost a state of grace. Our bodies probably misinterpret the athletic experience as life threatening and produce large quantities of endorphins.

The great athlete Pelé describes a peak-endorphin experience he had during a soccer game this way: "a strange calmness I hadn't experienced in any of the other games. It was a type of euphoria; I felt I could run all day without tiring, that I could dribble through any of their team or all of them, that I could almost pass through them physically. I felt I could not be hurt. It was a very strange feeling and one I had not felt before. Perhaps it was merely confidence, but I have felt confident many times without that strange feeling of invincibility."[9]

## Post-Event Peak

The post-event endorphin peak is far less dramatic, and occurs more often. It's a euphoric feeling that takes place after a hard workout or competition. Feeling no pain, you're filled with an overwhelming sense of contentment sometimes bordering on euphoria. Runners sometimes call this feeling "runner's high," but it is experienced by athletes in all sports. The feeling may last minutes, hours, or days. It may occur independently of any endorphin peak experienced during your workout.

# Smaller Amounts of Endorphins

As an athlete, you're more likely to experience endorphin peaks than a non-athlete. Still, these peaks occur rarely, maybe a few times during your life. Yet these peak experiences are important because they help us understand other, far less dramatic endorphin experiences. You probably experience, to a lesser degree, the effects of endorphins every time you work out. In situations involving less stress, you produce smaller levels of endorphins.

During massage, your body releases still smaller amounts of endorphins. This gentler dose is often enough to reduce pain and produce pleasure. Unlike other activities that release endorphins, self-massage gives each of us the ability to produce small quantities of endorphins at will, effectively alleviating pain and increasing pleasure. Each of us has this ability if we choose to use it.

# Endorphins and Massage

The quantity of endorphins released during massage probably varies roughly as a function of the stress released. Massage techniques that release more stress, such as those that release trigger points, probably release more endorphins. Massage techniques using acupressure, friction, and compression are also likely to produce endorphins. These massage strokes are described in Part II of this book.

It is likely that light gliding strokes release endorphins as well. These strokes give you a warm confident feeling while reducing pain and stress. The social dimension of this form of massage is clearly pleasing. You can see its effects in humans and other mammals; for example, the petting of dogs and cats and a mother touching a child's wound to make it better. Most of us like being touched, stroked, and hugged. Endorphins, at least in part, cause this good feeling when they're released into your bloodstream. You can create this feeling by using the light gliding strokes described in Chapter 8.

## Endorphins and Stress

All stress has the beneficial effect of producing endorphins, but not all activities that produce stress are beneficial. Some stressors are dangerous. In a world filled with stress, the choice of stressors is yours. You can choose beneficial stressors, activities that expose you to less risk of harm, or dangerous stressors, activities that expose you to more risk. For example, yoga is a beneficial stressor because it produces controlled degrees of physical stress, exposing practitioners to little risk of injury. Motorcycle racing may be considered a dangerous stressor because it produces uncontrollable degrees of physical stress, and exposes racers to a large risk of injury.

Self-massage is one of the most beneficial stressors because it gives you almost complete control of physical stress and exposes you to almost no risk of injury, making it one of the easiest and healthiest ways of creating stress to produce endorphins.

## In Summary

Endorphins are natural chemicals produced by your body to reduce pain and make you feel better. Self-massage is a healthful way to produce endorphins. Think of self-massage as an endorphin delivery system that you can activate anytime you like.

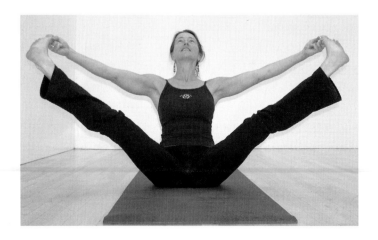

# Massaging Your Muscles

## How Massage Restores Your Muscles after Exercise

Your muscles are strong but delicate. They're made of micro-thin fibers that tear during a workout. Massage helps repair this micro damage more quickly by increasing circulation (which feeds and cleans muscles), realigning and restoring muscle fiber, and relieving muscle tension.[1]

## Facts about Your Muscles

Muscles are multipurpose marvels: they move you and heat you, weigh you down and lift you up. Muscles are the moving parts of the energy and information systems inside you. They transform electrical and biochemical energy into the mechanical energy that propels you. Seventy percent of the heat your body makes comes from muscles. Muscles account for 40 percent to 50 percent of your body's weight. They're what you eat when you eat meat. If you're lucky and take care of your muscles, they'll last a lifetime. If not, there's always golf.

You have two main types of muscles: skeletal and non-skeletal. Skeletal muscles are under your voluntary control and appropriately are called voluntary muscles. Non-skeletal muscles are everything else.*

---

*They include the muscles of the heart and the gut which operate involuntarily and ironically may control our greatest passions and most important decisions.

Your skeletal muscles move you on the playing fields and it's these muscles that you manipulate with massage. Your skeletal muscles are bound to your bones by tendons. They move your bones, so if your bones are shaking it's your skeletal muscles that are doing the shaking. You have about 620 skeletal muscles, all of which connect to the skeleton that lives inside you. Your skeletal muscles are strong but delicate. They're strong at the macro level but they tear at the micro level during workouts. All your skeletal muscles are made of the same magical stuff that's so mysterious not even the great drug companies can figure out how to make it.

## How Muscles Work

Your muscles are elastic. They contract and expand and then regain their shape. In fact, contracting and expanding is how they move your bones, and how your bones move the rest of you. Most muscles connect in opposing pairs on opposite sides of a bone. As one muscle in the pair contracts the other expands. In other words, when the muscle on one side of your bone shortens, the muscle on the other side lengthens. For instance, try bending your arm; as the muscle above your elbow contracts, the muscle below your elbow must expand. If it's not perfectly clear to you how every muscle in your body works and how your body keeps track of more than 600 of them expanding and contracting all the time, don't sweat it. Athletes have been performing miracles with their muscles for thousands of years without knowing exactly how they work.

Each muscle consists of many thin bundles of long skinny cells, called muscle fibers. Each muscle fiber comes in its own case or membrane. Think of a muscle fiber as being like a telephone cable containing many much-thinner fibers, called myofibrils, which are the width of fine thread. Within these ultra thin myofibrils are still thinner filaments made of protein.[2] The point of all this is that no matter how strong your muscles are, their very thin filaments can easily tear and get tangled up. And that's exactly what happens every time you work out.

All vigorous exercise produces small injuries—micro tears—to muscle fibers.[3] The more micro tears you have, the more likely you are to feel sore the next day. Whether these micro injuries grow into larger injuries or grow into stronger muscles depends on how well you recover before working out again.

In addition to causing micro injuries, exercise stretches your muscles unevenly, leaving them unbalanced. (Activities like sitting or sleeping also stretch your muscles unevenly.) Massage restores muscles to their balanced state. That's why it feels so good to massage your muscles after working out, or waking up, or, really, any time.

## Recovery

Massage helps your muscles recover, even after the toughest workouts. Using the three Rs of recovery, massage restores, relaxes, and relieves your muscles. Massage relieves muscle pain, restores circulation to your muscles, and relaxes muscle tension.

## Muscle Pain

Pain is one way your muscles have of telling you they need help. Massage provides that help: by increasing circulation, straightening muscle fibers, and releasing endorphins.

Massage forces fresh blood through your muscles removing the stagnant waste products that accumulate there and cause pain. By stroking your muscles, massage straightens muscle fibers that have become tangled, stuck together, and stretched out of shape. By applying direct pressure to knotted muscles, massage reduces pain by releasing endogenous morphine, your body's natural pain killer.

## Circulation

Massage pushes blood through your muscle fibers, feeding and cleaning them. Massage strokes force healthful oxygen-rich blood into your muscles and help remove the metabolic garbage that accumulates in your muscles during exercise. Increased circulation reduces your recovery time by boosting the speed at which your muscle cells are fed and cleansed.

## Muscle Tension

As you've probably noticed, your muscles sometimes feel hard and inflexible the day after a hard workout. By working directly on tense muscles, massage relieves muscle tension, which relaxes your body and mind. That may be why many athletes sleep better after massage.

At a micro level, muscle fibers tear and leak during hard workouts. These ultra thin fibers get stretched, pulled out of shape, and sometimes stuck together to form adhesions and knots. All this pulling, stretching, and knotting causes a chain reaction: tension in your muscle fibers causes tightness in your muscles, which causes a tension in your body and mind. By massaging muscle tissue directly under your skin, inelastic tissue recovers its soft elastic healthy state. And you feel better all over.

Massage also relieves muscle tension by heating your muscles. Because heat opens your blood vessels, it increases circulation. Heat also creates a feeling of well being. When it comes to your muscles, heat is sweet.

# Stretching Compared to Massage

To get a clearer idea of how muscles work, let's compare stretching a muscle to massaging it. Static stretching has become popular in the last thirty years. Athletes use it before and after workouts. Some athletes find static stretching helpful; others find it painful. To effectively stretch a muscle, you must lengthen the muscle to feel a not-quite-painful tension, and hold it there for anywhere from ten to sixty seconds.

When performing a static stretch, you stretch your muscle fiber lengthwise. Like stretching rubber bands, stretching a muscle elongates the muscle fibers. Each muscle contains many bundles of muscle fiber. Because the many bundles of fiber in a muscle are stretched as one, the stretch is limited by the least flexible muscle bundle. Thus, the only part of your muscle to get stretched is the least flexible part. Massage lets you stretch different parts of the muscle independently. The stretch that massage gives not only feels good but can be targeted to the exact place that will do you the most good.

With static stretching, the stretch usually pulls the muscle one way, lengthwise. It's more difficult to stretch it crosswise. With massage it's easy to stretch your muscles lengthwise, crosswise, and otherwise.[4] To get a feel for the difference, try stretching the muscles in your forearm between your wrist and your elbow by bending or twisting your wrist. Now try massaging the same muscles. Use your thumb and four fingers to apply pressure and roll the same muscles you stretched. Try keeping your thumb on the same area of skin while moving the muscle underneath. Move your thumb lengthwise, crosswise, clockwise, and counter-clockwise. The massage has a multidimensional effect while the static stretch has a limited effect. That's one of the differences be-tween massaging a muscle and stretching a muscle.

Because with static stretching you're often using the force of your body, the stretch is likely to be more powerful than the stretch you get with massage. The stretch from massage is likely to be gentler and more precise.

To perform static stretching effectively, the right stretching technique is crucial.[5] Athletes must learn and use the proper technique. Most authorities agree, if stretching is not done correctly it can cause more harm than good.[6] Self-massage is far less technical and is extremely safe. It's hard to do more harm than good with self-massage.

## In Summary

Muscles are strong but delicate. During workouts, they suffer micro tears and trauma. Massage helps muscles heal from these injuries.

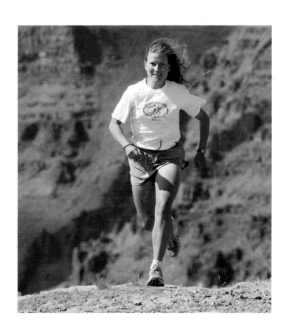

# Muscles & More

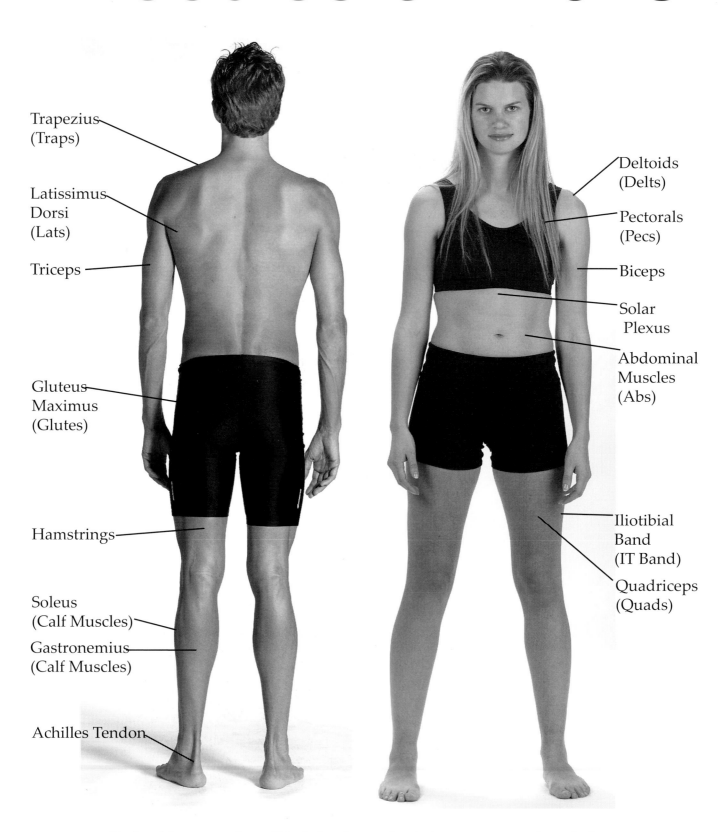

Trapezius
(Traps)

Latissimus
Dorsi
(Lats)

Triceps

Gluteus
Maximus
(Glutes)

Hamstrings

Soleus
(Calf Muscles)

Gastronemius
(Calf Muscles)

Achilles Tendon

Deltoids
(Delts)

Pectorals
(Pecs)

Biceps

Solar
Plexus

Abdominal
Muscles
(Abs)

Iliotibial
Band
(IT Band)

Quadriceps
(Quads)

Each of the more than 600 skeletal muscles living in you can benefit from
massage. Some of the most needy muscles and more are named above.

# PART II

# Learning
# Self-Massage

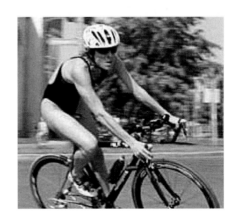

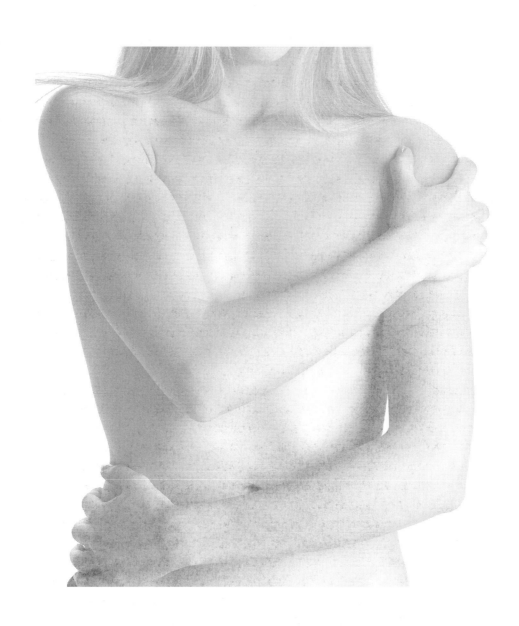

# Introduction to Part II

Welcome to Part II. This is the hands-on, learn-by-doing, I-can't-wait-to-get-my-hands-on-myself, part of the book. It's where you actually learn self-massage.

In Chapter 8, you'll learn the *seven simple massage strokes* that make up a great massage. Chapter 9 offers rules and tips for applying the strokes, and a word about pain. In Chapter 10, you'll practice applying the strokes to each part of your grateful body, after which, in Chapter 11, you'll learn *when* to apply the strokes. Chapter 12 touches on improvisational massage. Once you've completed Part II of this book, all you'll need is a little practice and a great massage will never be farther away than your fingertips.

There are only three basic moves to learning self-massage: *gliding*, *pressing*, and *pulling*. First, you *glide* your hand over your skin. Second, you *press* directly on your skin to compress your muscles. Third, you grip a muscle and *pull* it. That's it! That's all there is to it. Six of the seven massage strokes* are just variations on these three fundamental moves. If you can learn to glide, press, and pull, you can learn to give yourself and anyone else a great massage.

If you follow the simple instructions in this part of the book, you'll begin to think with your hands while learning self-massage. You'll also discover a new way of relating to your body. As you practice, you'll improve; as you improve, you'll feel even better. By making self-massage a regular practice, it'll become a healthy habit that will last a lifetime.

---

*And the seventh is something you've been doing your whole life in one form or another.

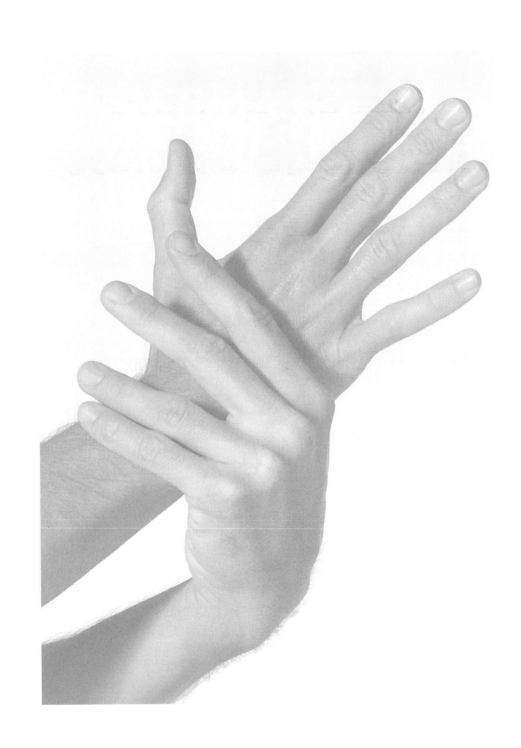

# 8

# Seven Simple Massage Strokes

## That Will Put the Power in Your Hands

*"What we have to learn to do, we learn by doing."*—Aristotle

To give yourself a great massage, you only need to know seven simple massage strokes:

**1. Gliding**

**2. Squeezing**

**3. Squeezing & Rolling**

**4. Pressing**

**5. Pressing & Rolling**

**6. Drumming**

**7. Rock & Rolling**

Each stroke is easy to learn and fun to do. If you learn the strokes on each page before turning to the next page, by the time you reach the final page of this chapter you'll be on your way to a lifetime of great massages.

Let's begin.

# STROKE # 1: GLIDING

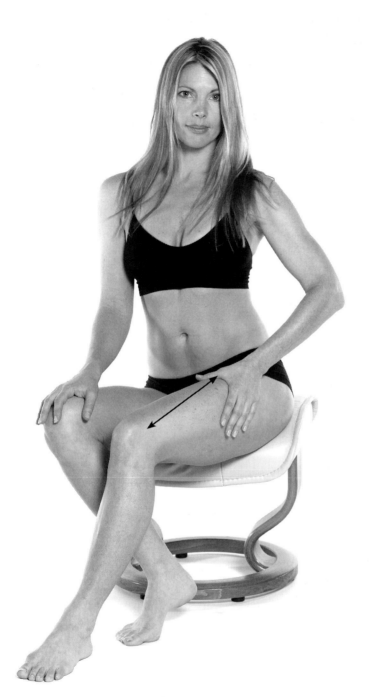

**Try It:** Try seven light *gliding strokes* up and down your upper leg. Slightly vary the location and intensity of each stroke. Then try it on your other leg.

**Purpose:** *Gliding* is a good beginning for every massage. It warms your skin and sends a message to your body that a massage is coming.

**Stroke Description:** Glide your hand over your skin.

**Note:** Massage therapists call this stroke by its French name *effleurage*, which means gliding or skimming.

**Tips:** Volume, velocity, and intensity are three variables you can use to change the effect each stroke has on you.

**Volume:** Try covering more skin with each stroke by spreading your fingers wide or make a "V" between your thumb and index finger.

**Velocity:** Try varying the speed of your strokes.

**Intensity:** Try varying the pressure applied to each stroke.

**Tips:**
- Apply greater pressure when stroking toward your heart and lighter pressure when moving away from your heart. Applying pressure in the direction of your heart assists your blood on its way back to your heart.
- Alternately, relax and flex the muscles you're massaging.

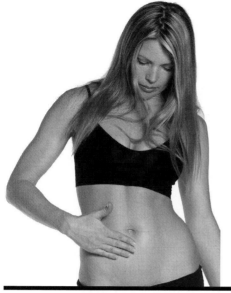

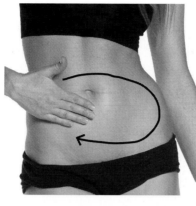

**Try It:** Try a series of seven circular *glides* on your abs. Vary the volume, velocity, and intensity of each stroke. It should feel pretty good. If it doesn't, maybe you've got the wrong set of abs. Try massaging your own belly.

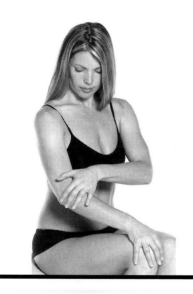

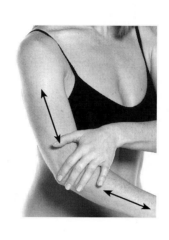

**Try It:** Move your hand over your entire arm. Do a series of seven *glides* on your arm from your wrist to your shoulder. Vary the volume, velocity, and intensity of each stroke. Direct your attention toward your arm. Then try it on your other arm. How does it feel?

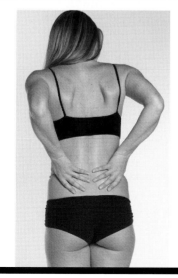

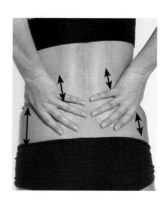

**Try It:** This stroke requires some reach. It's best to stand up for it. Do a series of seven short *glides* on your lower back. Vary the length and intensity of each stroke. The purpose of this stroke is to warm your lower back, and to reintroduce your hands to a part of your anatomy they haven't been to in a while.

Turn the page when you're comfortable doing all the strokes on these two pages and are ready to go deeper into massage.

# STROKE # 2: **SQUEEZING**

Squeezing is pleasing.

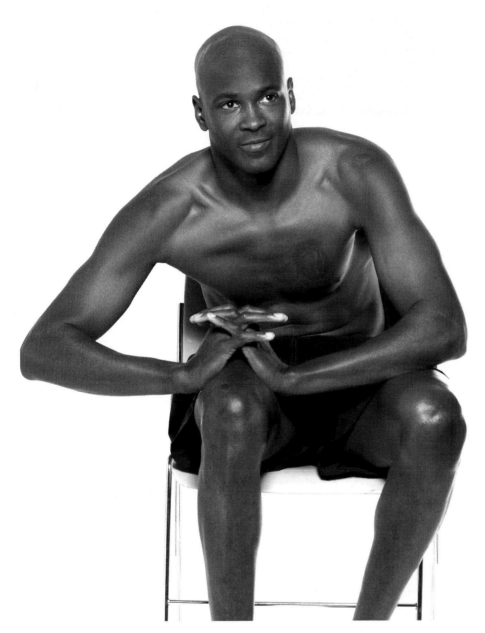

**Try It:** Interlace your fingers. Rest the heels of your hands on either side of your thigh and squeeze your hands into your thigh muscles (quads). Try seven slow quad *squeezes*. Slightly vary the location and intensity of each *squeeze*. Now, try it on your other leg.

**Purpose:** *Squeezing* warms muscles, increases circulation, and speeds recovery.

**Stroke Description:** Squeeze the muscle.

**Note:** Massage therapists call this stroke *compression*.

**Tips:**
- Focus your awareness deep inside the muscle you're squeezing.
- Squeeze your muscles, not your bones.
- Grab your whole muscle—squeezing is not pinching.
- Close your eyes and feel deep within yourself. Self-massage can be a meditation.
- Try turning off the language center in your brain and allow your hands to communicate directly with your body.

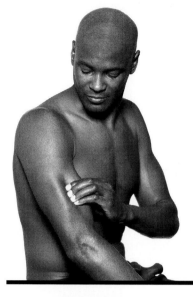
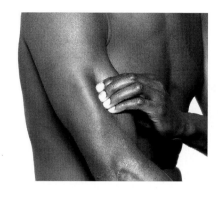

**Try It:** Squeeze your biceps. You don't have to take off your shirt, but it's best to massage bare skin. Try a series of seven *squeezes*. Relax your arm. Slightly vary the location and intensity of each squeeze. Close your eyes and focus your attention deep inside the muscle you're squeezing. Then try it on your other arm.

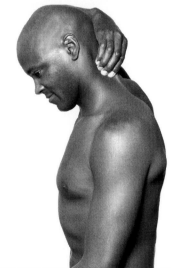
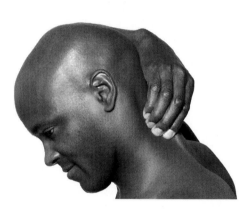

**Try It:** Try a series of seven slow *squeezes* on the back of your neck. Lay the heel of your hand on one side of your neck and your fingers on the other side. Squeeze your hand and fingers against your neck. Slightly vary the location and intensity of each *squeeze*. Relax your neck muscles while squeezing. You might try this same stroke using your other hand.

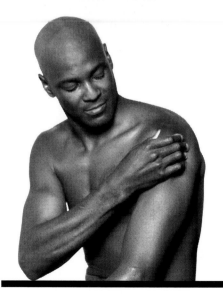
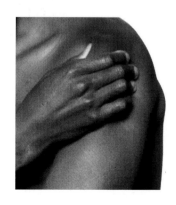

**Try It:** Let your thumb and four fingers grip and squeeze the muscle. Try a series of seven *squeezes* on your shoulder muscles (deltoids). Slightly vary the location and intensity of each *squeeze*. Relax your shoulder. Then try it on the other shoulder. How does it feel?

Turn the page when you feel comfortable squeezing your entire body.

# STROKE #3: SQUEEZE & ROLL

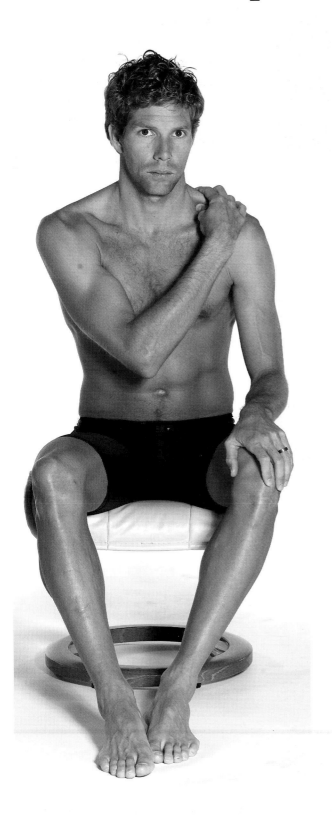

**Try It:** Squeeze and roll the muscle between your neck and shoulder. It's hard to tell from the photo that he's doing anything other than squeezing the muscle. But you should in addition to squeezing your muscle also pull or roll the muscle between your fingers. Try it. First squeeze the muscle, just like you did on the previous page. Then pull it a little and roll it in a small circle or back and forth. Try seven slow *squeeze & rolls* on your trapezius muscle varying the intensity of each stroke. Let your muscles relax.

**Purpose:** *Squeezing & rolling* increases your circulation and warms your muscles. It also gives your fingers a good workout.

**Stroke Description:** This is a two-step stroke. First squeeze the muscle just like you did on the preceding page. Then pull the muscle and roll it between your fingers. The rolling motion moves the muscle up and down; it pulls the muscle away from your body. It's similar to kneading dough.

**Note:** Massage therapists call this stroke by the French word *petrissage*, which means kneading.

**Tips:**
- To completely relax, try lying on your back.
- Focus your full attention on your muscle as it moves around between your fingers.

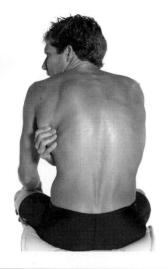

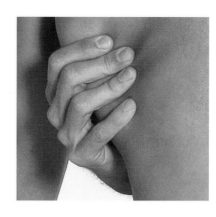

**Try It:** The *squeeze & roll* may be the most challenging of the seven massage strokes. But you can do it. Just squeeze the thick muscle that makes up part of the back of your armpit. Try a series of seven *squeeze & rolls*. Relax your lats. Then try it on your other side.

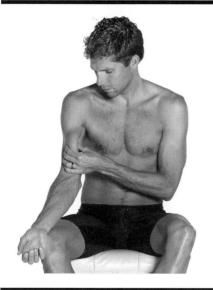

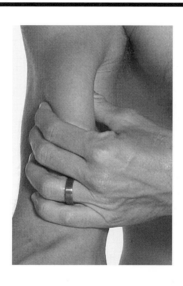

**Try It:** Grab hold of your biceps and roll them. Try a series of *squeeze & rolls*. Continue the rolling until it feels good. It will eventually feel good. Slightly vary the location with each series of strokes. Then try it on your other arm. Try it on your triceps.

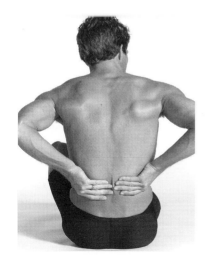

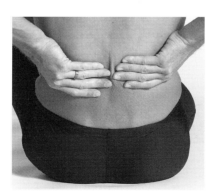

**Try It:** The muscles in your back are tough to squeeze and roll. Try a series of seven *squeeze & rolls* on your low back. Slightly vary the intensity of each stroke. Relax your back. If nothing else, it gives your arms a good stretch and is a good way to get more blood flowing to your back.

Turn the page when you feel comfortable doing all the *squeeze & rolls* shown above and three more of your own invention.

# STROKE # 4: **PRESSING** or Poking

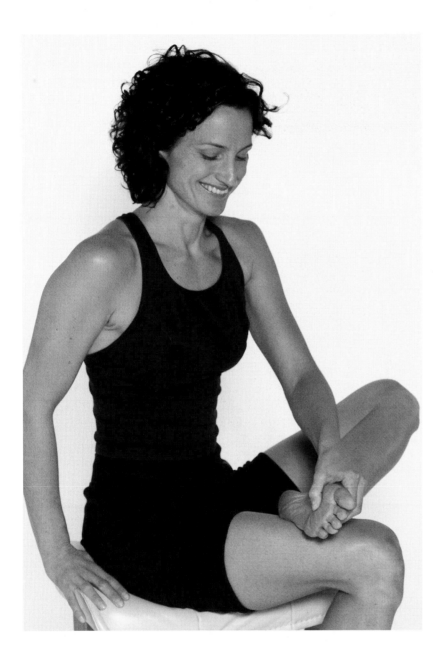

Poking is stoking.

**Try It:** Take off your shoes and socks and give your foot a poke. Press your thumb into the bottom of your foot and your other four fingers into the top of your foot. Try seven slow *presses*. Experiment by varying intensity and moving your fingers slowly over your foot. Try it on your other foot.

**Purpose:** The *press* and *poke* are powerful strokes because they activate acupoints, trigger trigger points, jump-start circulation, and send endorphin cocktails flowing to every cell.

**Stroke Description:** Press or poke a muscle into the bone, using one or more fingers, fists, or elbows. Hold the press from one to thirty seconds. A *press* is just a slow *poke*.

**Note:** Massage therapists call this stroke *compression*.

**Tips:**
• Press perpendicular to your muscle.
• Focus your awareness deep inside the muscle that you're pressing.

**Intensity:** Varying the intensity of a stroke is the most effective way to vary the effect of the stroke. Vary the intensity of a *press* stroke by pressing harder. An intense *glide* is just a light *glide* with extra pressure applied.
• You can apply extra pressure with your hand, or use your body's weight to exert more intensity.
• To get a more intense stroke, lean your body in the direction of the stroke.

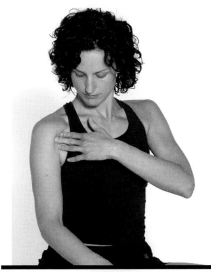

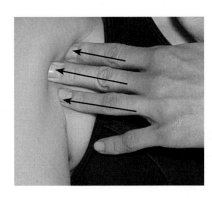

**Try It:** Try a series of seven *presses* to your delts. Use a single finger *press;* then try using multiple fingers. Relax and vary the location and intensity of each *press.* Try it on your other shoulder.

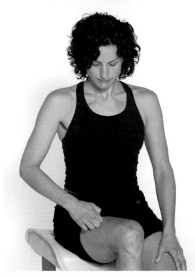

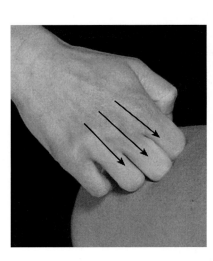

**Try It:** Make a fist and press or poke your knuckles directly into your quads. Try a series of ten *presses.* Vary the location and intensity of each *press.* Alternately relax and flex your leg muscles. Then try your other thigh.

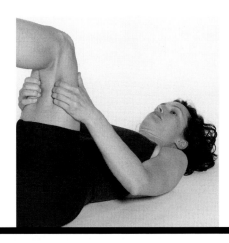

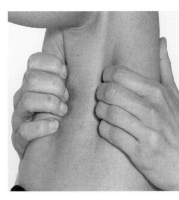

**Try It:** You may do this seated or lying on your back. Try a series of ten *presses* to your hamstrings using four fingers. Vary the location and intensity of each *press.* Relax your leg muscles. Use one or two hands. Then try it on your other leg.

Turn the page when you've tried all the *presses* above and have *poked* every part of your body that needs *poking.*

# STROKE # 5: PRESS & ROLL

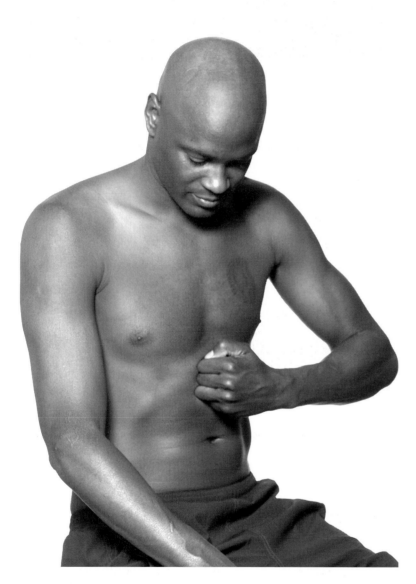

**Try It:** Starting at your solar plexus *press & roll* your abs. Perform a series of small circular rolls with your fist moving clockwise, until you've covered your entire belly with your fist. Slightly vary the intensity of each stroke. Alternately, relax and flex your abs. Feel the difference between *pressing* and *pressing & rolling* your abs. It's like night and day.

**Purpose:** *Pressing & rolling* activates acupoints, triggers trigger points, jump-starts circulation, and sends endorphin cocktails cruising to stimulate every cell in your body.

**Stroke Description:** The *press & roll* is the *press* with a twist. Press the muscles into the bone to compress them. Then roll or rotate your press. Your fingers, elbows, or fists can be used to press and roll your muscles.

**Note:** Massage therapists call this stroke *friction*. It can be used for deep tissue massage.

**Tips:**
- Press your fingers against the muscle, then roll your fingers, so that you can feel the muscle circling beneath your skin.
- *Press & roll* perpendicular to the muscle. Focus your awareness deep inside the muscle that you're rolling.

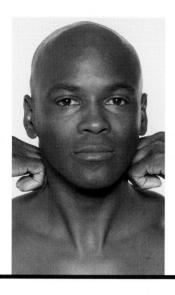

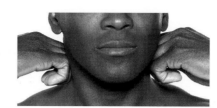

**Try It:** Press the sides of your neck with your fists, then roll your fists in small circles on your neck muscles. Twist your fists at your wrists. Relax your neck. Vary the pressure. Move in small circles around your neck until you've covered both sides of your neck and your neck is warm.

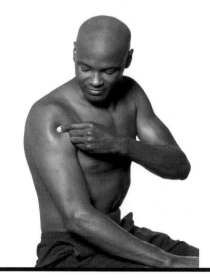

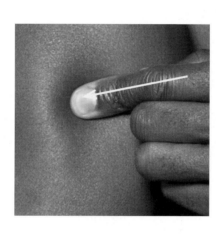

**Try It:** Give your shoulder a *press* with one finger. Then roll that finger on the muscle and feel the muscle roll with your finger. Try a series of seven *press & rolls* on your shoulder muscles. Vary the location and intensity of each stroke. Try *pressing & rolling* with multiple fingers. Then try it on your other shoulder.

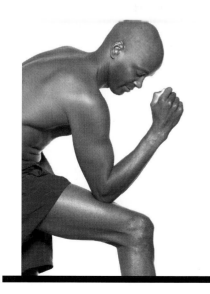

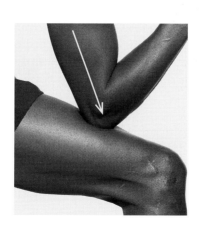

**Try It:** Try a series of seven *press & rolls* using your elbow on your upper thigh. Your elbow brings more intensity to the stroke than your fingers or fists. Vary the location and intensity of each stroke. Relax your quad muscles. Try it on leg #2.

Turn the page when you're confident that you can *press & roll* any muscle that lives inside you.

# STROKE # 6: DRUMMING

The language of the body is rhythm.

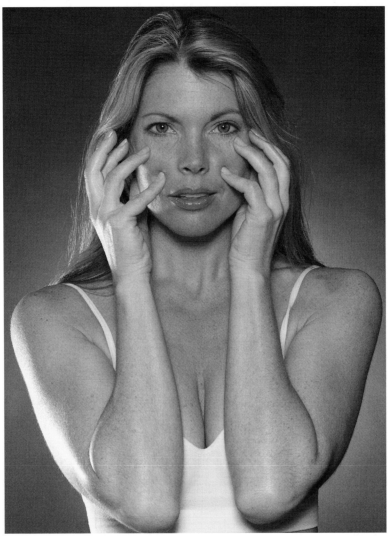

**Try It:** Lightly drum your fingertips on your face. Vary velocity, intensity, and location until your fingers have touched every beautiful space on your face.

**Purpose:** *Drumming* is an energizing stroke, used to get you moving.

**Stroke Description:** Lightly drum or tap your hand on your body. By varying the part of your hand *drumming* your body, the feeling of the stroke changes. Some examples are open flat hand, open cupped hand, side of hand, fist, knuckles, side of fist, and fingertips.

**Note:** Massage therapists call this stroke *tapotement*. It means drumming.

**Tips:**

• Keep it light.

• Play your body like you would a sensitive drum; listen and feel each stroke.

• Focus your full attention on how each stroke feels.

• Surrender to the stroke.

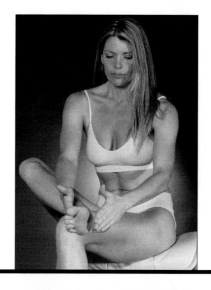

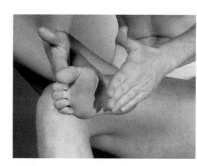

**Try It:** Take off your shoes and socks. Then begin to *drum* your foot with your hands. It should feel good. Vary the location and rhythm of each stroke. Let every muscle in your foot soften and relax.

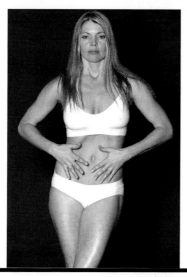

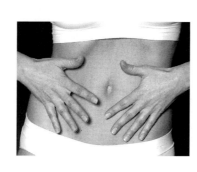

**Try It:** Play your abs like you would a drum. Gently stroke out a rhythm. It's a nice feeling and a nice sound. *Drum* your abs and chest. Vary the location and rhythm. Relax your abs and pecs. Have fun with your drum.

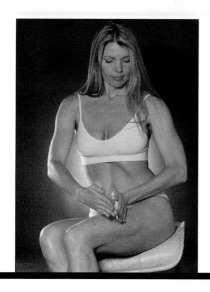

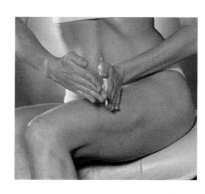

**Try It:** *Drum* your quads. Use the sides of your hands. Slightly vary the location of each stroke. Let your leg relax. Focus on the rhythm and feeling of each stroke.

Turn the page after you've tried *drumming* your entire body and are ready to *rock & roll*.

# STROKE # 7: ROCK & ROLL:

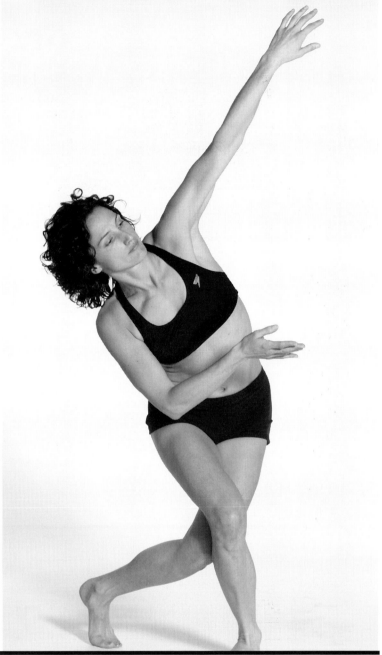

**Try It:** Play your favorite dancing music and let it play you.

**Purpose:** To massage your internal organs and increase your circulation. To move your entire human being: body, mind, and spirit. To warm, ready, and strengthen your muscles. *Rock & roll* is a great way to prepare for any activity.

**Stroke Description:** Dance to rock & roll music or any music that moves you. Most people don't think of dancing as a massage stroke, but it is. Dance massages everything that lives inside you and increases your circulation.

**Note:** Massage therapists may not use this stroke, but you should.

# DANCING

*"Wake it and shake it."* —Ken Keesey

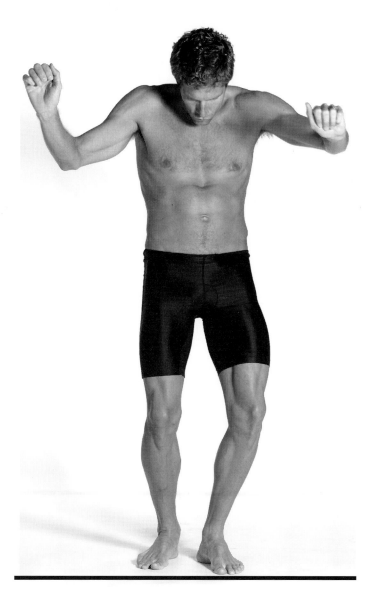

**Tips:**
- Play the music loud enough to feel it inside you.
- Turn your brain off and focus your attention inside your body.
- Glide your hands over your body as you dance.
- Let the music move you.
- Play music that touches you and has a driving rhythm; *Drums of Passion* by Babatunde Olatunji may do it for you.

Turn the page when you're all shook up and ready to go.

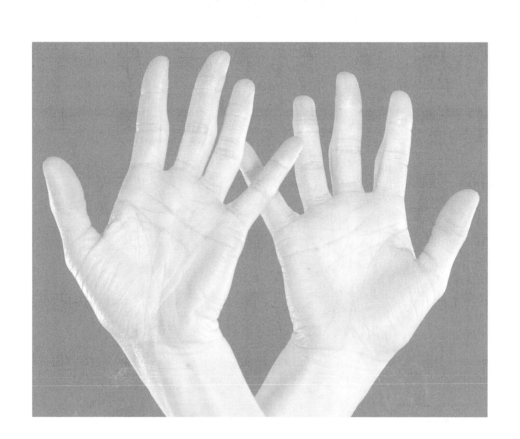

# 9

# Rules, Tips, and Pain

Ten Rules, Five Tips, and a Word about Pain

## Ten Rules

1. Trust yourself.
2. Devote your full attention to feeling each stroke.
3. Massage muscles, not bones.
4. Bare skin massages best.
5. If it feels good, it's good; if it feels bad, it's bad.
6. Improvise and invent; every massage is an experiment.
7. Turn your brain off and let your body guide your hands.
8. Experiment by relaxing, lengthening, and flexing the muscles you're massaging.
9. If injured, get help from a qualified healthcare provider.
10. It's your body: You get to make the rules.

# Five Tips

1. How to identify areas that need your attention:

   - Your muscle feels tight when you touch it.
   - Your muscle feels tight or stiff without touching it.
   - Your muscle feels hard compared to its twin muscle on the opposite side of your body.
   - A portion of your muscle or tissue is hard compared to the muscle surrounding it.

2. To improve the quality of your massage, close your eyes.

3. If you have a question about how to do any of these strokes, consult our web page, SelfMassageForAthletes.com, or ask a massage therapist. Going over these strokes with a massage therapist may be helpful.

4. To give yourself a relaxing massage, lie down and completely relax your body, especially the muscles that you're massaging.

5. Self-massage is a way of making your body happy, and if your body is happy the rest of you will be too, because you and your body are one.

# A Word about Pain

It's unlikely that you will hurt yourself practicing self-massage. But you may experience a little pain. Some athletes think of pain as a more intense form of pleasure. And if that works for you and the pain does you no harm, that's fine. But be aware that pain in and of itself is not a good thing when performing massage on yourself or someone else.

Most athletes understand there are two kinds of pain: unfortunately, both are painful. There is creative pain and destructive pain. Creative pain leads to improved health. Destructive pain does not. Creative pain is the pain associated with birth, therapy, adaptation, and improvement. After the pain subsides, it often results in a pleasurable feeling. Destructive pain is unhealthy pain: pain for its own sake. It is harmful pain, pain that usually arrives by accident or from an opponent.

It's often difficult to distinguish creative pain from destructive pain. If something you are doing feels like it is damaging or hurting you, it probably is. Stop doing it. If your massage is causing you pain and you can't determine whether it's the healthful or harmful type of pain, you should stop and consult a healthcare professional.

# 10

# A Sample Massage

## Learn by Doing a Full Body Massage

The secret of self-massage, if there is one, is learning to think with your hands. It's that simple. You don't have to know anatomy or the names of the 600+ muscles living in your body to give yourself a great massage. If you want you can call them all "Bob."

In this chapter, you'll learn to think with your hands. As you apply the seven simple massage strokes you learned in Chapter 8, you'll learn to trust your hands and let your fingers take direction directly from the part of your body they're massaging. By turning off your brain and letting your hands think for you, you may discover that they have an energy and intelligence all their own. They understand your body in a way your brain never will.

The more attention you direct to an area of your body, the more benefit it will get. Your muscles will tell you where to massage, how hard they need to be worked, and how long to continue massaging. Listen to your body.

As you massage sore muscles, try different strokes, speeds, and intensities. Use the variations that feel best. Don't worry about how much time it takes. Continue working the muscle until you no longer feel you're benefiting.

You can massage each part of your body by following the order of pages in this chapter. We begin with the hands, then go to the arms, shoulders, neck, face, chest, abdomen, back, feet, lower legs, upper legs, and end with the butt. In that way you'll get a full body massage. Alternatively, you can begin by massaging the parts of your body that most need it.

Remember to let your body direct your hands. Every massage is an improvisation.

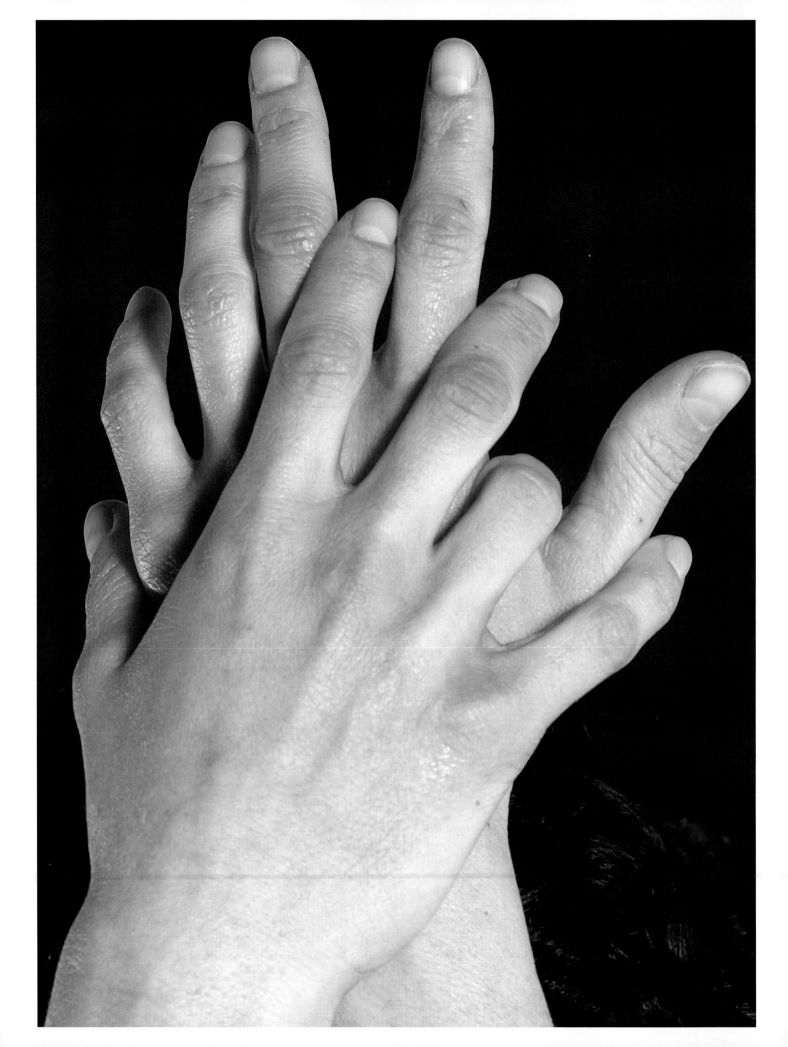

# Hands

With practice, your hands can develop into fine massage tools. They have the power to go deep into your muscles. They're sensitive and precise; each fingertip contains thousands of sensory receptors. They're flexible enough to fit your body like a glove. They're smarter than you think, and will get better and better at making you feel better. All they need is practice.

Self-massage keeps your hands healthy. Every time they give you a massage, they get a massage. Massage exercises each of the thirty-seven skeletal muscles that live in your hand. It keeps them strong and responsive. Your hands work best when treated well. Let them massage each other once in a while and they'll pay you back in everything they do.

## Massage Your Hands

**Gliding:** It's good to begin every massage with warm hands. *Gliding* your hands together will do just that. *Glide* or rub your hands together.

• Do fronts and backs.

• Rub knuckles together.

**Squeeze** the area between your thumb and index finger.

• Use one hand to grip and pull each finger on your other hand.

**Press** your right thumb into the front of your left hand and the four fingers of your right hand into the back of your left hand. *Press* your thumb toward your four fingers. Vary location. Switch hands and repeat.

**Drum:** Lightly clap, slap, and drum your hands together, fronts, backs, and sides.

Tip: Let your hands listen to and be directed by each other. After a few massages you can abandon the above directions and let your hands take over.

**Time: Take two to three minutes to massage each hand, or however long you want.**

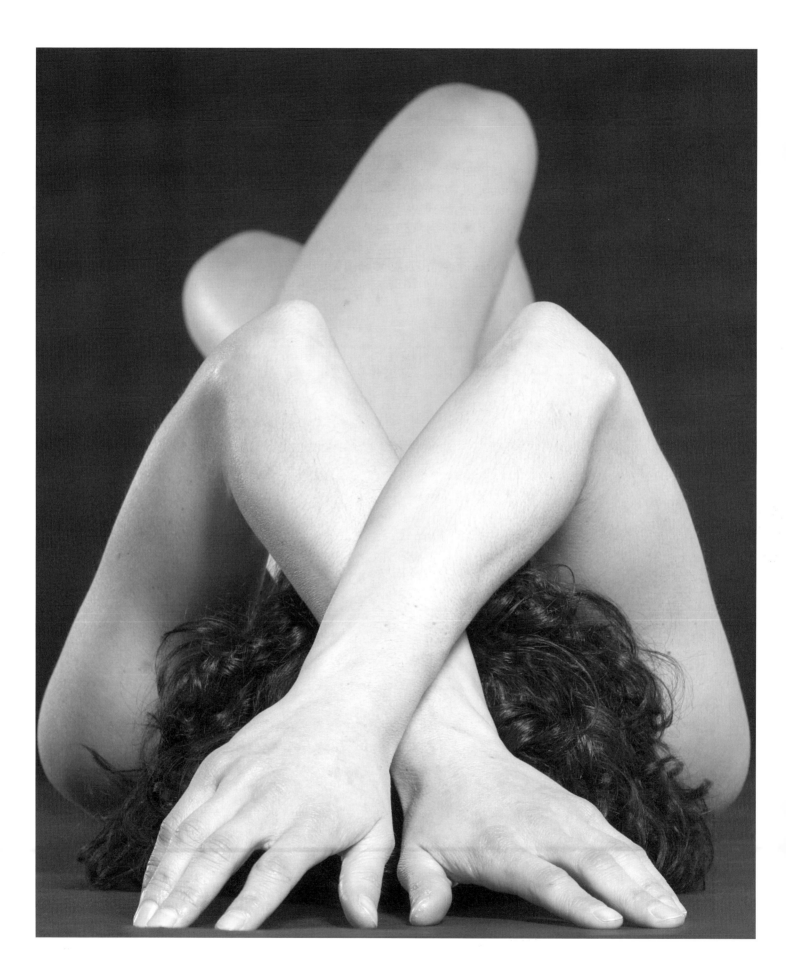

# Arms

Massaging these long muscular levers juices every living thing between your shoulders and fingertips. By revving your circulation, massage can revive your tired aching arms.

Arms are designed for movement. They throw, push, swing, stroke, pull, and lift. Active healthy arms are mostly muscles: triceps, biceps, and more. It is the aches and pains in our muscles, especially near our joints, that make us seek the solace of massage. If you overuse your arms, the muscles surrounding your wrists, elbows, and shoulders may be stiff and sore. To keep your arms swinging and performing their best, self-massage works wonders.

---

## Massage Your Arms

**Glide** your hands up and down your arms, experimenting with velocity and intensity. Turn off the language center in your brain.

• Cover your entire arm with between five and fifty strokes. Continue until both arms feel warm.

• Try *gliding* your knuckles over the front, back, and sides of your lower arms.

**Squeezing:** Try a few series of *squeeze* strokes beginning at your wrists and ending at your shoulders. Vary velocity and intensity.

**Squeeze & Roll** the muscles in your upper arms.

**Press & Roll:** Gently *press & roll* the muscles in your lower and then upper arms.

**Drum:** Perform a set of ten to twenty *drum* strokes up and down your arms.

**Tip:** After massaging each part of you, take thirty seconds to relax and breathe deeply to fully feel the effect of the massage.

---

**Time: Give two or three minutes to massage each arm, or however long you need.**

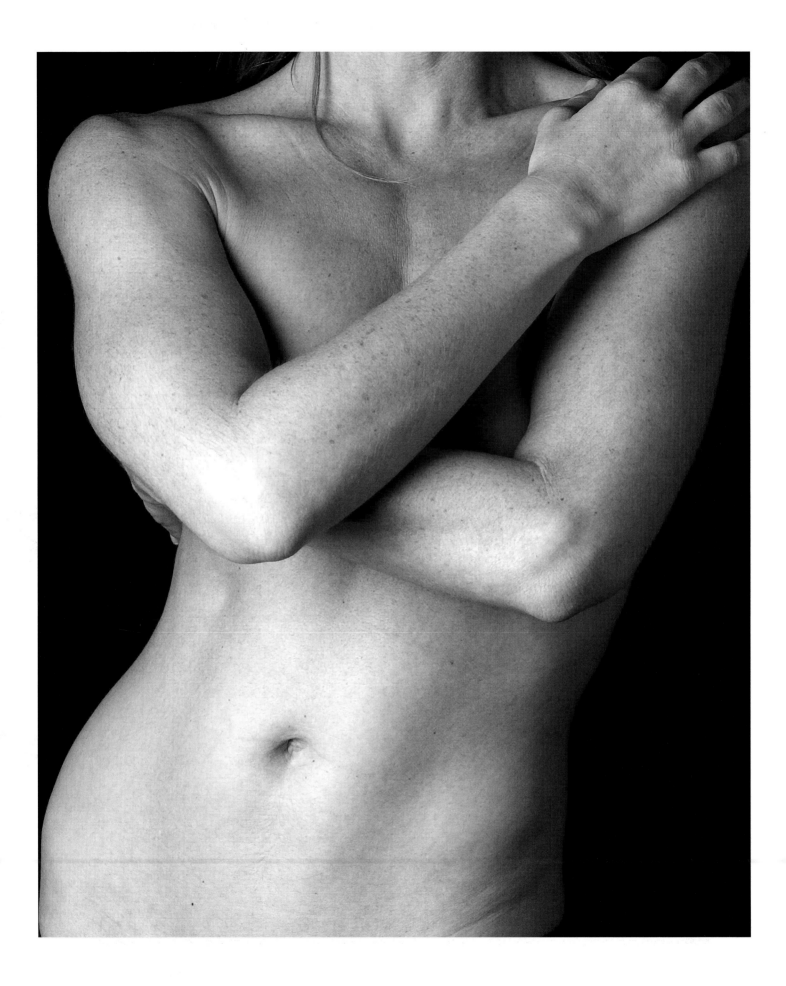

# Shoulders

Sports that involve swimming, lifting, throwing, and swinging put a strain on the muscles surrounding your shoulders, especially your deltoids and the four muscles of the rotator cuff. While highly mobile, shoulders are prone to injury. With overuse, they grow stiff, tending to get old before the rest of you. Massage may be the fountain of youth they need.

Your shoulders' biggest job is to direct your arms, keeping them as stable and dynamic as your sports require. To do their job, your shoulders are made of ball-and-socket type joints and millions of muscle fibers needed to move those joints through their paces. Massage keeps your shoulder muscles moving, healthy, and young.

## Massage Your Shoulders

**Glide** your open hand from the base of your neck to your upper arm to warm your shoulder with about ten strokes of varying intensity.

**Squeeze** the muscles surrounding your shoulder joint, using all five fingers; vary location slightly with each *squeeze*. Let your shoulder relax.

**Squeeze & Roll** the muscles, in back, between your shoulder and neck (trapezius muscles) using four fingers and a thumb.

• To relax your trapezius lay on your back.

**Press or Press & Roll** the muscles surrounding your shoulder joint using one, two, or all five fingers. Massage the front and back of your shoulder, paying attention to the muscles surrounding your shoulder joint.

• Focus all your attention on the muscles you're massaging.

**Drum** your hand on your shoulder and feel the stroke penetrate your muscles.

**Tip:** To completely relax your shoulder try lying on your back.

**Time: Take three or four minutes to massage each shoulder, or as long as it takes.**

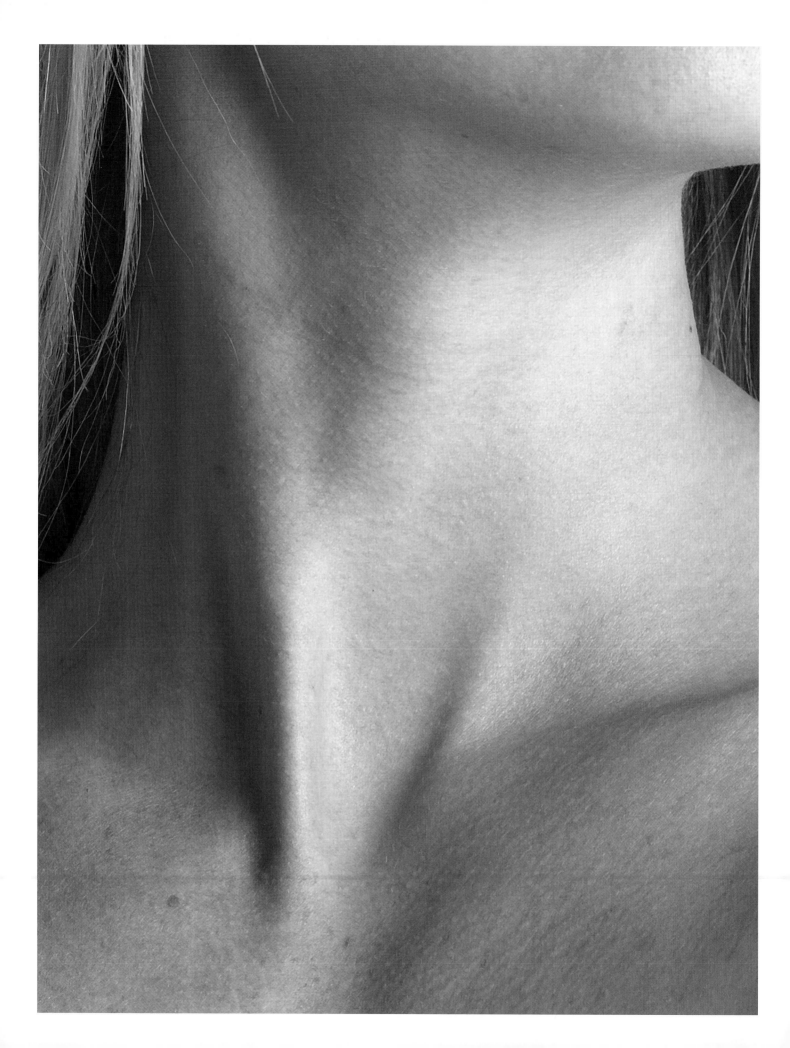

# Neck

There are two types of athletes: those who have suffered from sore stiff necks, and those who will suffer from sore stiff necks. Your neck has the unenviable job of balancing and catering to a demanding sixteen-pound weight all day and into the night. So your neck muscles have to be strong, tolerant, and responsive.

An athlete's neck faces special risks. It's responsible for keeping your head from getting hit by flying objects, fists, balls, sticks, pucks, and whatever else comes flying at it. As an athlete, your neck must be powerful and flexible. A good massage will not only help make your neck strong as an ox's but loose as a goose's.

---

## Massage Your Neck

**Glide** both hands over your neck until it is warm.

**Press & Roll** using both hands on either side of your neck. Place all five fingers from your left hand on the left side of your neck and all five fingers from the right hand on the right side of your neck. Roll your hands varying velocity and intensity.

• Feel deep inside your neck and relax it completely.

• Use all ten fingers to gently cover your whole neck, the muscles in front from your collarbone up to your jaw, and in back up to your skull.

• You may want to try this same stroke with your knuckles, *pressing & rolling* on either side of your neck.

**Drum** your neck lightly using your fingertips or open fists.

**Tip:** The secret to a great neck massage is to surrender, relax every muscle in your neck, and let your hands do their stuff.

**Time: Devote three to five minutes to massage your neck, or however long you need.**

---

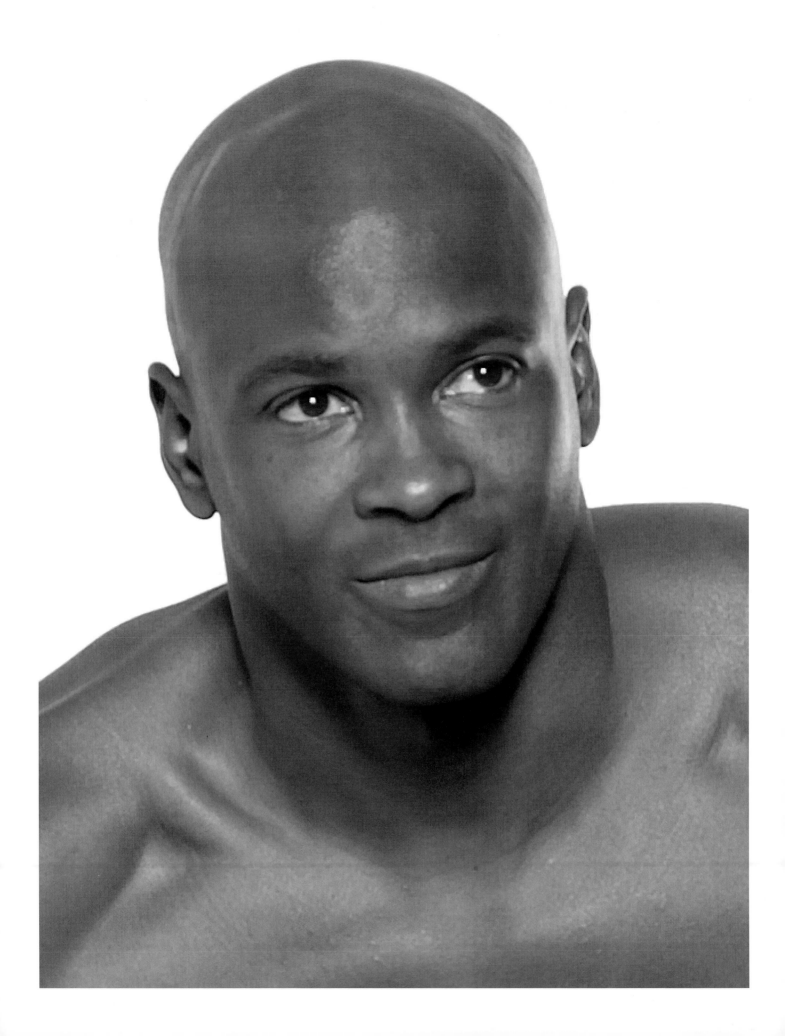

# Face

A facial massage does more than make you look good. It makes you feel good and perform better. More than any other part of you, your face represents who you are. It's your communication center. It inspires love and communicates beauty. It reveals and conceals emotions. It reflects health and well being. Traditional Chinese and Japanese medicine use facial appearance as an important indicator of health. A facial massage will not only improve the way you look and feel, it will improve your entire sensory system.

Your face is home to your sense organs—sight, smell, hearing, taste, and touch—all live here. That may be why your face is so sensitive to massage. Massage helps all your senses function optimally, irrigating your sense organs with new blood, nutrients, and oxygen. Because all your senses are crucial to your success as an athlete, by giving them frequent massage, you'll notice a difference in how you look, feel, and perform.

---

# Massage Your Face

**Glide** both hands lightly over your entire face and scalp.

• Feel every muscle in your face relax.

**Squeeze** gently with both hands all over your head, further warming your face and scalp.

• Pull, tug, and twist your ears gently to get the blood flowing.

**Press** your face and scalp with a single finger or multiple fingers.

• Use three fingers to *press* underneath your chin.

**Press & Roll** with both hands on either side of your face. Do your entire face until it feels warm and ready.

**Drum** your face and scalp with your fingertips.

Tip: Do it again but this time let your hands be directed by your face, not this book.

Time: Massage your face for as long as it takes.

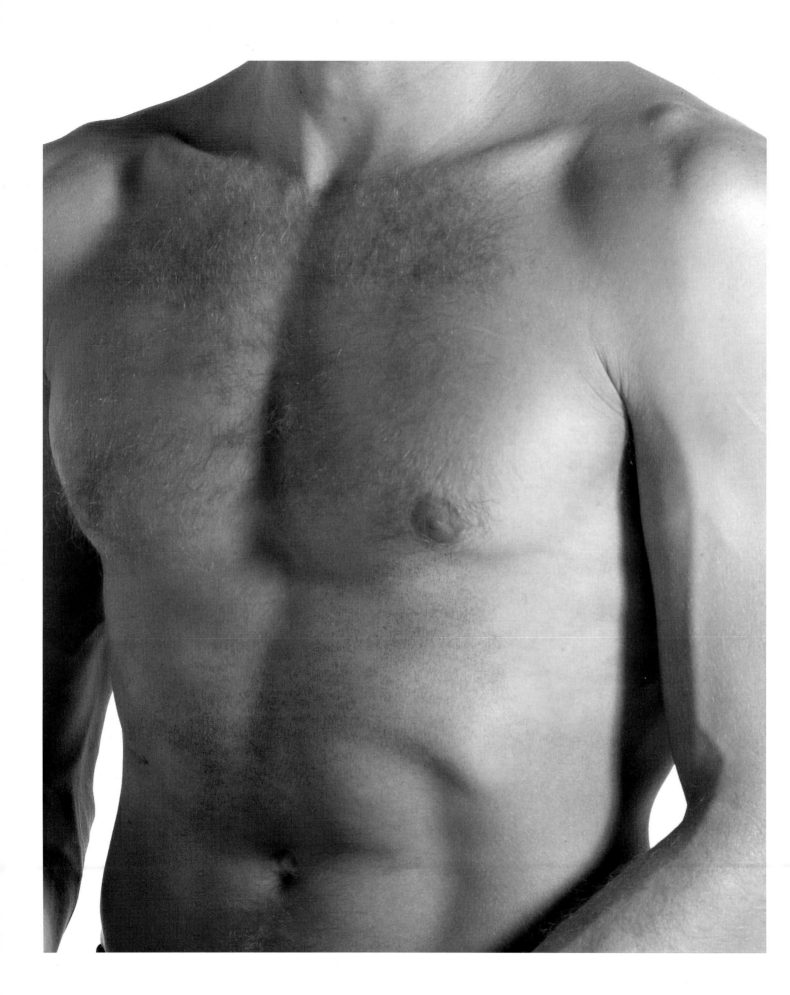

# Chest

Your chest is home to your heart and lungs. Each works better after a hearty massage. The chest also houses your pectoral muscles which are especially useful in racket sports. Pecs play an important role in arm movement and stabilization. They get ample play in any activity that employs a lot of upper-arm muscles like swimming, throwing, rowing, climbing, and swinging a bat, racket, or club. If you do any of these things often, you'll do them better with frequent massage. The best reason to massage your chest? It feels good.

## Massage Your Chest & Ribs

**Glide** your hand in a circular motion over your entire chest until you feel a warmth penetrate your chest and hand. *Glide* your hand over your ribs and lats.

**Squeeze & Roll** your pecs and lats.

**Press** directly with both thumbs on each side of your chest and ribs, releasing those endorphin cocktails.

**Press & Roll** using five fingers from each hand directly on your chest and between your ribs.

**Drum** your fists against your chest, like Tarzan.

**Tip:** Focus your intent and breath into the muscles you're massaging.

**Time: Devote five minutes to massaging your chest and ribs, unless it takes longer.**

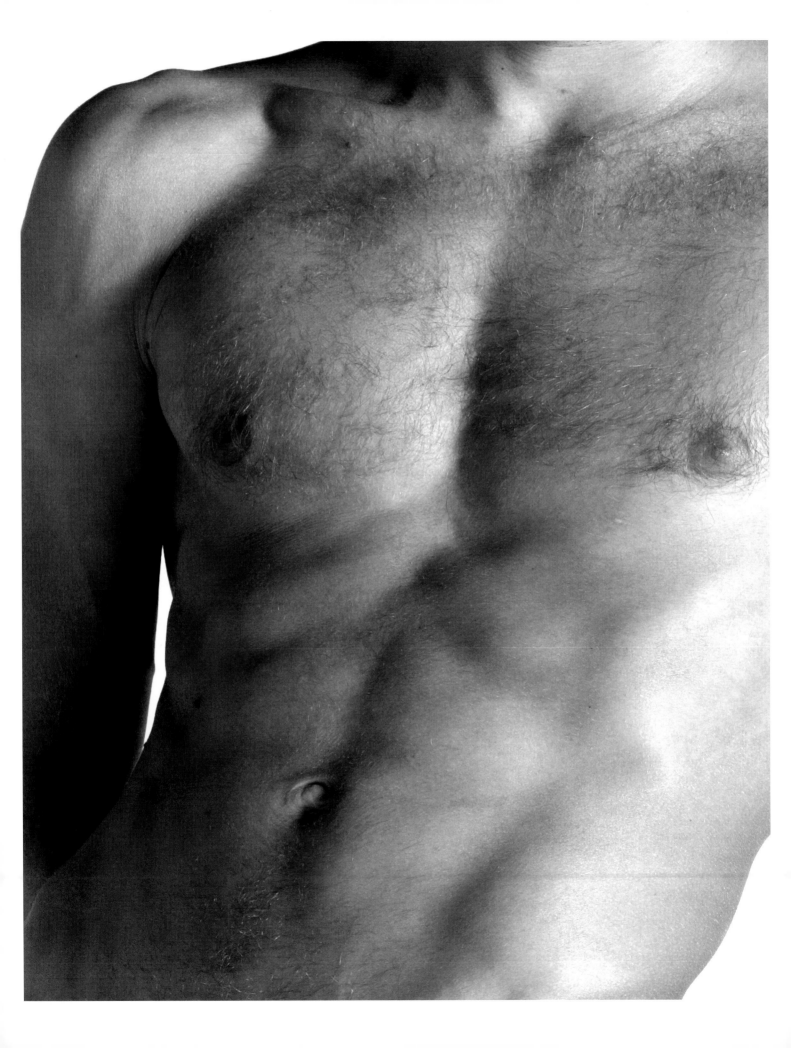

# Abdomen

Your abdomen is home to your intestines, stomach, liver, gall bladder, kidney, spleen, and pancreas. All these organs benefit when you massage the skin and muscles above them. In addition to these organs, a complex network of nerves, called the solar plexus lives in your abdomen. If you massage the area between your rib cages, these nerves will relax your entire being.

Finally, the abdomen sports our only set of *superstar* muscles, regularly featured on magazine covers and in their own infomercials. They are known, throughout the English-speaking world, by one name: **Abs**. These muscles support your internal organs and help you breathe. They are your core; they stabilize you, and keep your top half from bumping into your bottom half. Your abs may not always be as visible as you would like, but they're always there for you, supporting and helping you.  They are surprisingly responsive to massage.

# Massage Your Abs

**Glide** your hand lightly round and round over your abs so you can feel them warm and relax. Breathe through your nose and into your belly.

- Alternately flex and relax your ab muscles.

- Try interlacing the fingers from both hands together and *glide* the heels of both hands around your abs.

**Press & Roll** using four fingers over the muscles in your abs.

- Alternately flex and relax your ab muscles.
- Experiment by *pressing & rolling* with different finger combinations and parts of your hand.
- Place your fist over your solar plexus and gently roll your fist.

**Drum** your abs with open hands, varying the rhythm of your stroke.

**Tip**: Massage with the intent of healing the part of your body you're massaging.

**Time: Massage your abs three to five minutes, or until you're ready to move on.**

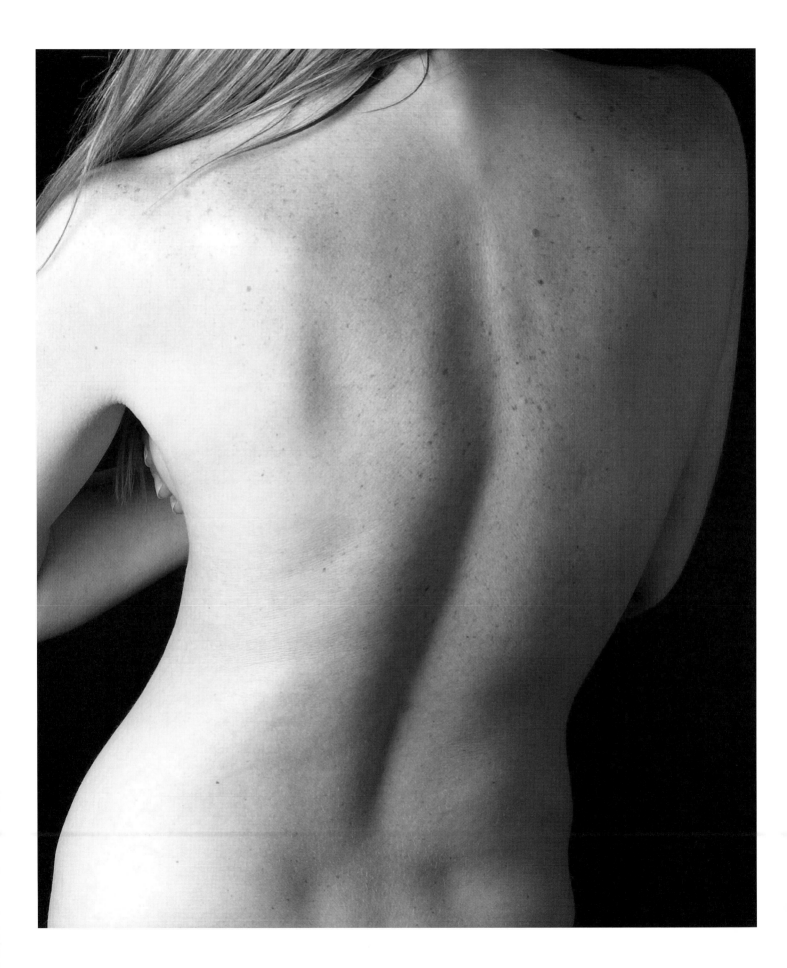

# Back

Sixty percent of adults suffer from back pain each year. More workout days are lost to back issues than any other health problem, except death. Almost all sports, from pole-vaulting to chess, put a strain on your lower back. Massage relieves that strain and reduces your chances of injury.

Each of the many muscles lining your back has an important job. They stabilize, support, and move your spinal column. They provide strength and flexibility to your core. They help move your shoulders, arms, and neck. Back muscles get sore from all this work and need massaging. Unfortunately, being back muscles, they're located in back and may be hard to reach.

While it takes practice, patience, and imagination, you can learn to massage your back. Don't worry about learning to massage the parts of your back you can't reach; just learn to massage the ones you can.

## Massage Your Back

### Full Back:
**Glide** your bare back against the back of a large comfortable chair or carpeted floor.

• Gently roll your back in a swaying motion; close your eyes.

### Upper Back & Lats:
**Glide** your hand, reaching around over your shoulder as far as is comfortable. Try supporting your elbow with your free hand.
**Press & Roll** using three fingers while supporting your elbow with your free hand. Reach over your shoulder and then go under your arm to your lats and back ribs.

### Lower Back:
**Glide** both hands on both sides of your lower back.
**Press & Roll** using all 5 fingers.
**Drum** your lower back with the front of your fist.

**Tip:** The above techniques are at best a good stretch. For a great back massage see the massage tools in Chapter 16. They can help you massage your entire back, honest.

**Time: A good back massage can take all day but try to limit yours to ten minutes.**

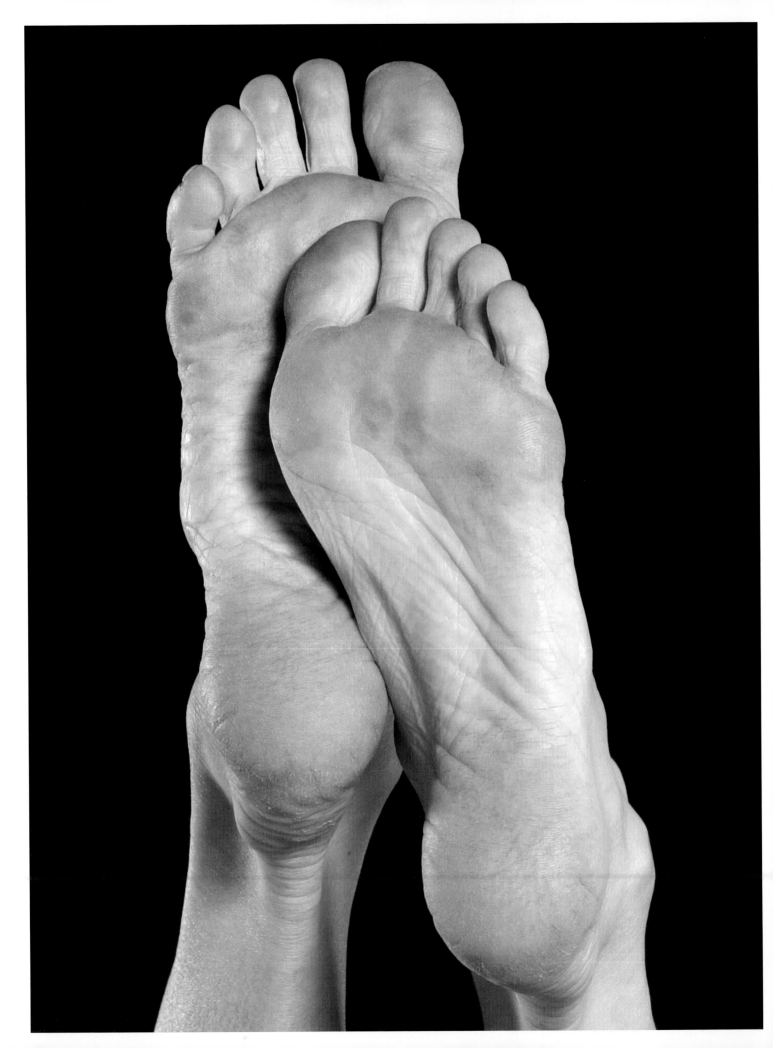

# Feet

Your Feet Take a Licking and Keep on Kicking

There's a fine line between exercise and self-abuse, and nowhere is that line more often crossed than with the feet. Our feet balance us, carry us, and move us. In return, we stuff them into socks and shoes, and command them to take us everywhere. Our feet don't like this treatment. They are more sensitive to pain and overuse than we imagine.

Millions of years ago, before shoes and socks, the feet, like the hands, ran around naked and helped our human ancestors explore their world. To aid this exploration, the feet, like the hands, are endowed with thousands of nerve endings. That's why feet are so sensitive and appreciative of massage. They have the sensitivity of our hands but are treated like our butts.

Thirty-three skeletal muscles and thousands of sense receptors make your foot extremely receptive to massage. A foot massage is a giant step toward a healthier, happier athlete. Give your feet frequent massage and they'll take you wherever you want to go.

# Massage Your Feet

**Glide** both hands over your foot for warmth.

• Try *gliding* your knuckles over the bottom of your foot.

**Squeeze** all five toes together a few times, then roll your whole foot at the ankle, relaxing and surrendering to the sensation.

**Squeeze & Roll** each toe, gently pulling, twisting, and stretching it.

**Press** using your thumb on the bottom of your foot and four fingers on the top. Press the thumb and fingers toward each other.

**Press & Roll** using that same thumb on the bottom of your foot.

**Drum** your foot with open hands, then stretch your toes and relax.

**Tips:**
• For best results while massaging, keep your feet bare and your eyes closed.

• For a discussion on the risks of massaging someone else's feet, see *Pulp Fiction*.

**Time: Give each foot a three or four minute massage.**

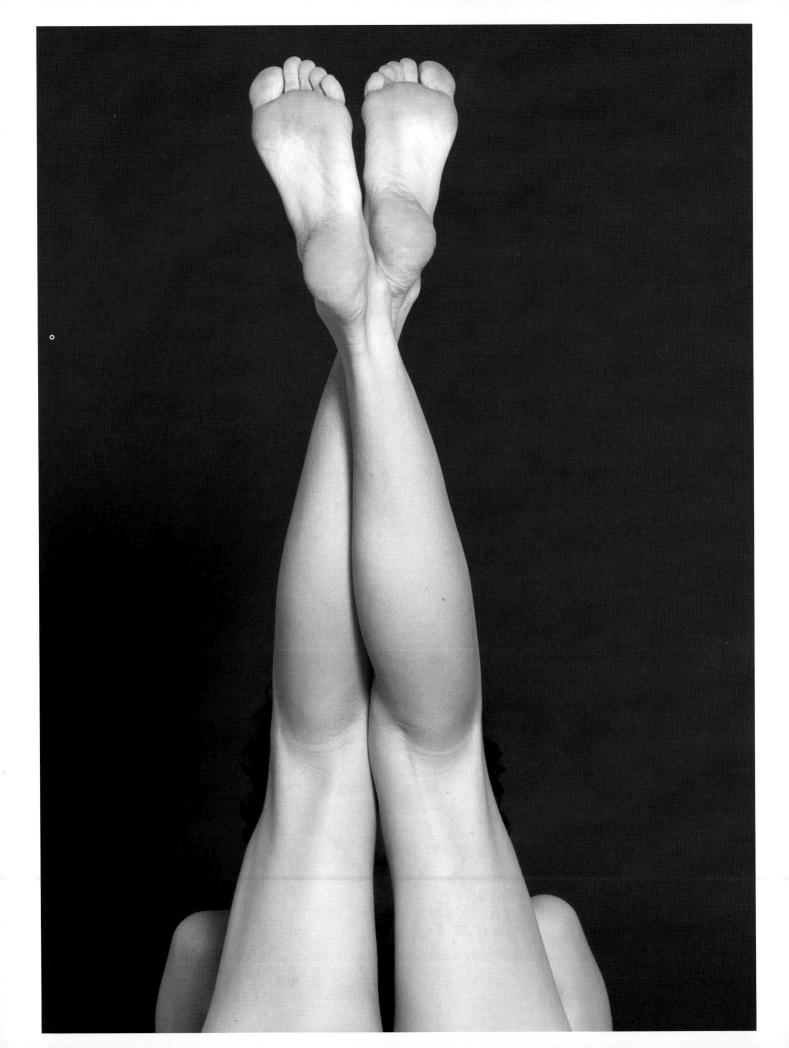

# Lower Legs

Touch the part of your leg that lives between your heel and knee. It's home to your calf muscles which live in the back, and your soleus muscles which live on the sides. Both calf and soleus muscles move and flex your foot which keeps you from falling over.

   If you're a doctor, you know there are hundreds of things that can go wrong with the muscles in your legs. If you're a runner, you've probably experienced every one of them. Try something that can make every muscle in your lower legs feel good.

## Massage Your Lower Leg and Knee

**Glide** both hands up and down your lower leg to warm the area from your heel to your knee. If you're sitting or lying down, cross your legs, resting the leg you're massaging on top of your other knee.

- Continue until your skin is warm and ready.

- Try circling your hand gently over your knee to get it hot.

**Squeeze** the muscles between your heel and knee in the back of your leg. Begin with your Achilles tendon and work your way up.

**Squeeze & Roll** your calf muscles between both hands.

- Interlace the fingers from each of your hands, place them on your knee, and gently *squeeze & roll* the muscles surrounding your kneecap.

**Press & Roll** the muscles on the outsides of your calf, called the soleus. Try using a fist or four-finger *press & roll* stroke.

- Use both hands on either side of your leg to compress the muscles living in the sides of your leg.

- *Press & roll* the muscles surrounding your kneecap; use all ten fingers simultaneously.

**Tip:** To relax all the muscles in your leg, lie on your back.

**Time: Give each lower leg a three to five minute massage.**

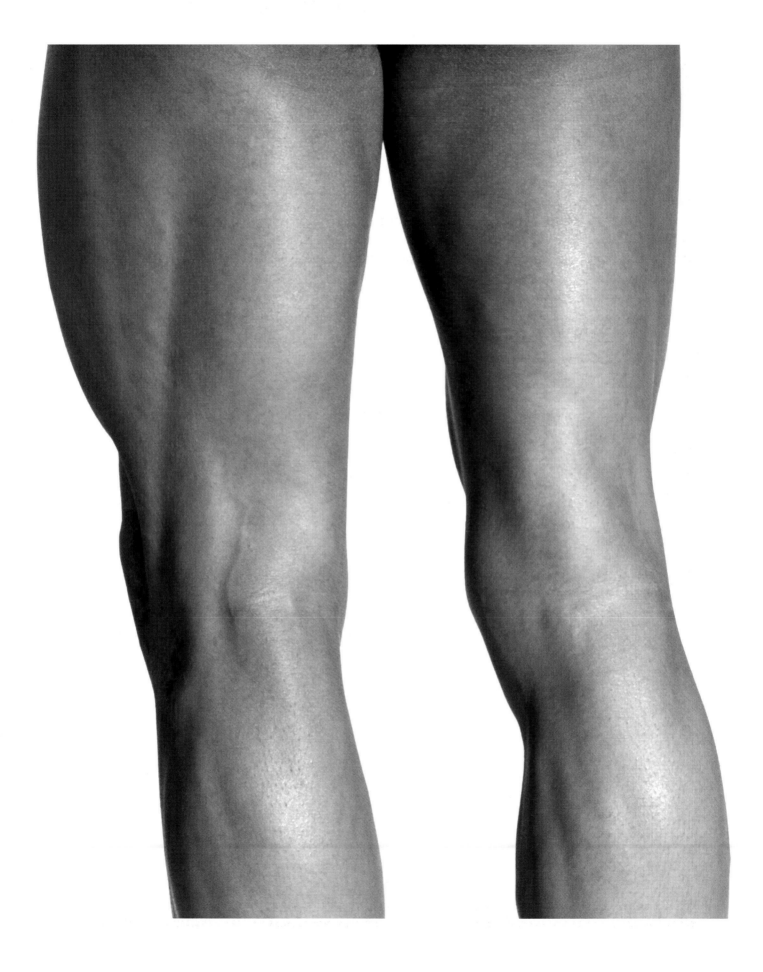

# Upper Legs

Your upper and lower legs account for about half your body's height. Blood traveling from your feet to your heart could use a hand fighting gravity, especially after a tough workout. Massage provides that hand.

The two big sets of muscles living in your upper legs are your hamstrings and quadriceps. Both muscle groups move your knees and lower legs. Your hamstrings are three muscles in the back of your thigh. They bend your knees and extend your hips. Your quadriceps are four muscles inside the front of your thigh. They extend your legs and straighten and stabilize your knees. They're crucial for walking, running, and standing. If you use your quads a lot, you should massage them a lot.

If your sports involve significant running or the use of your upper-leg muscles as in boarding, cycling, skating, surfing, or skiing, you know what to do.

## Massage Your Upper Legs

**Glide** your hands up and down your upper leg from your knee to your butt to heat them up. If you're sitting or lying down, cross your legs, resting the heel of the leg you're massaging on top of your other knee.

**Squeeze:** Interlace the fingers of your hands together and, using the heels of your hands, *squeeze* your quads and hamstrings.

**Press** up and down your quads using both fists. Then try *pressing* with just your fingertips. Finally, use your fingertips to *press* your hamstrings.

**Press & Roll** using both fists up and down your quads.

- Use your elbows on your quads to go deeper as needed.

- *Press & roll* your fingers straight up into your hamstrings, using both hands.

- Using your fist on the sides of each leg, *press & roll* your way up from your knee toward your hip and then do it again

**Drum** your upper leg with your fists to energize your legs.

Tip: To fully relax the muscles in your upper leg, lie on your back.

**Time: Give each upper leg a three to five minute massage.**

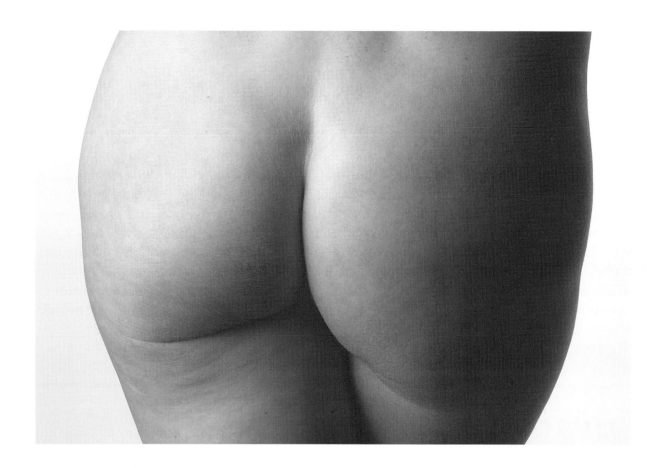

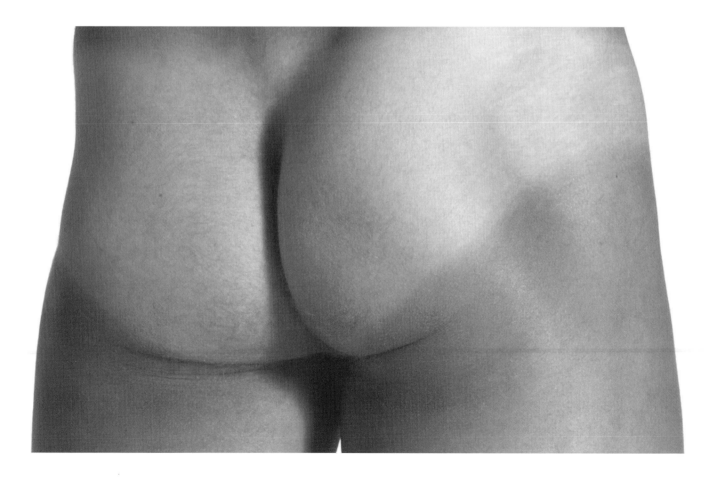

# Butt

*"No matter which way you turn your butt is always behind you."*—Francois Truffaut

Your butt is supported by your gluteal muscles—glutes for short—which cover the back of your pelvic bone and are attached to your thighbone. Your glutes do more than just sit around waiting for something to happen. They're the largest muscles in your body for a reason. They move your hip joints and thighs, which move your legs, which move the rest of you.

The glutes are subject to overuse injuries by all athletes. But no athlete is at greater risk from overusing their glutes than golfers. Whether it's from the rigorous training they do on the 19th hole or from driving those golf carts, is hard to say. Whether you golf or not, a glute massage is a wonderful thing. Give your glutes a treat, massage your seat.

---

# Massage Your Butt & Hips

Note: You can't take this sitting down. Lie on your side to relax your glute & hip muscles.

**Glide** your hands lightly over your glutes and hips.

**Press** your glutes and hip muscles using four fingers or use a massage tool like the Dolphin, Body Back Buddy,® or TheraCane.™

**Press & Roll** those glutes. You can try this with your fists, but will probably find it much more effective to use a massage tool, as mentioned above.

**Drum** your open hands on your glutes and hips. Use the heels of your hands or your fists.

• This may feel surprisingly good and make you wonder why spanking has gotten the reputation it has.

Tips:

• Relax and breathe deeply into your nose, and out your glutes.

• You need a massage tool to penetrate the extremely large muscles that are your glutes.

**Time: Give each side five to ten minutes of massage as needed.**

## Ten Minutes per Day for Three Weeks

Now that you've massaged your entire body, it's time to plan a practice. Recognizing that most people don't have unlimited time to learn self-massage, here's an easy way to get started. Practice self-massage ten minutes a day for three weeks. Pick a time during the day that's convenient for you, either first thing in the morning or before going to bed, or while counting the many reasons you're grateful you don't play golf. The goal is to be consistent; it doesn't matter when you practice massage, but that you do it at the same time every day.

Begin by massaging that part of you that feels like it needs it most. Use each of the strokes described in this book to allow your hands to get comfortable with them. Then turn off your brain's language center, and let your hands communicate directly with your body.

Three weeks is a good length of time in which to become comfortable using all seven self-massage strokes. It lets you enjoy the many benefits of self-massage, while reinforcing the habit of practicing the techniques. During this three-week learning period, you may find you want to massage longer than ten minutes a day. Good, go as long as you feel you want to, but practice at least ten minutes every day.

During the first three weeks, you'll begin to enjoy the health, athletic, mood, and recovery benefits of self-massage. By the end, you'll either continue using self-massage on a daily basis because you enjoy its benefits and can feel them working all day or you'll modify your practice to meet your personal needs. For example, you may decide to practice massage only before or after workouts, or when you experience muscle soreness. Alternatively, you might find you use self-massage when you're stressed, depressed, or anxious, or when your immune system needs a boost.

If you continue practicing daily, don't feel confined to just ten minutes. Most people like to go longer. Just listen to your body.

## In Summary

Give yourself ten minutes a day, and in three weeks, you'll be comfortable using self-massage whenever you need it.

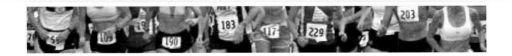

# 11

# When To Use Self-Massage

Your Pre-Workout Massage
and Recovery Massage

Athletes usually hire massage therapists when pain begins to erode performance or when they have a little extra money and time. That's probably not often enough. The best time to get a massage is when you need one. With self-massage, you can get relief anytime you want it: before, during, or after a workout.

## Pre-Workout Massage

The purpose of a pre-workout massage is to get you ready for your workout or competition. Depending on your athletic needs on a particular day, you may want to be stimulated or relaxed. With self-massage you can do either by fitting your stroke to your need. Brisk and intense strokes are stimulating. Slow, low-pressure gliding strokes are relaxing.

The purpose of the warm-up massage is to prepare your body, mind, and spirit for action. The pre-workout massage warms your skin and muscles and reduces the likelihood of injury.

How much time you spend on your warm-up massage depends on need. Most athletes devote between five and ten minutes, but don't let that stop you from spending an hour if that's what it takes to meet your needs.

Your strokes should be light to moderate in intensity. To begin, glide your hands over your entire body to warm your skin. Press harder to warm up the major muscle groups you will use during your workout. Devote special attention to any stiff muscles. Always warm up your neck because it invariably needs it.

Your warm-up massage may be performed any time before your workout or competition. Whenever you have time, and your body feels you need it. If you do it far enough in advance of your workout, it becomes a recovery massage.

## Recovery Massage

Your post-workout or recovery massage should be done in time to help you recover, usually within twenty-four hours of a workout or competition.

The purpose of a recovery massage is to relieve your sore muscles after hard exercise and help you recover faster for your next workout. The recovery massage is intended to soothe and relax you.

Like a warm-up massage, your recovery massage should take as long as you need. Most athletes devote about thirty to forty minutes to it. But again, if it takes longer to meet your needs, take longer.

Use any intensity that helps you feel better. It will probably be deeper and more intense than a pre-workout massage. You may want to concentrate on the primary muscles used during your workout.

Use whatever sequence of strokes your body wants. If your body's indifferent to where you begin, try the following sequence:

- Begin with hands, arms, neck, shoulders, chest, stomach, face, head
- Next: toes, feet, legs, thighs, butt
- Last: back (see the massage tools described in Chapter 16)

## A Hard Day's Night

Self-massage can also be used in the mornings as a way to wake up and recover from a "good night's sleep." Sleeping can be surprisingly hard on your body. A good massage in the morning can do wonders to help you recover from even the most strenuous night's sleep.

# 12

# Improv Massage

## Every Massage Is an Improvisation

No matter how many times you use self-massage, you'll never massage the same body twice. That's because your body is always new, constantly changing, expanding, shrinking, growing, reaching, and improving. As your body changes, your needs change. No two massages will ever be the same. Your body's needs change too fast for that.

Improvisation is the key. Now that you've learned the seven simple massage strokes, described on the preceding pages, and explored each part of your body, you can improvise with confidence. Your hands will learn to sense your changing needs and satisfy them. Your hands will adapt to tailor your massage to meet those needs. Every time you perform a massage, you'll feel your hands doing something new.

Use the massage strokes that make you feel best. By practicing the strokes in this book, you will learn the skills required to do just that. Through practice, you'll develop techniques to meet your changing needs and give yourself the best possible massage every time.

As you've probably discovered, self-massage is 50 percent art, 50 percent science, and 100 percent you. It's an art in which you are both the artist and the canvas. It's a science in which you are both the scientist and the experiment. And always, it is an improvisation.

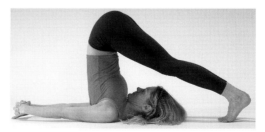

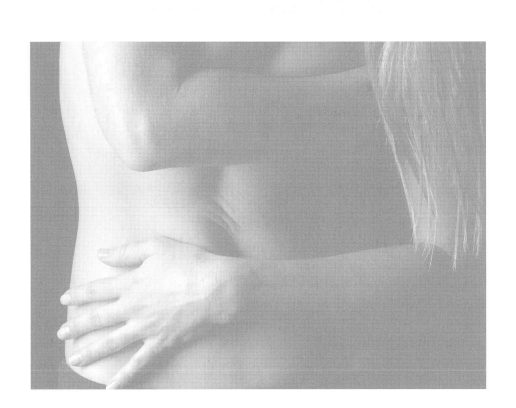

# PART III

# Going Deeper:

## Getting More
## from Your Massage

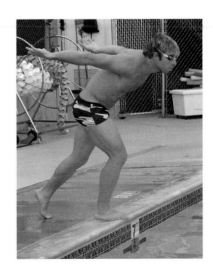

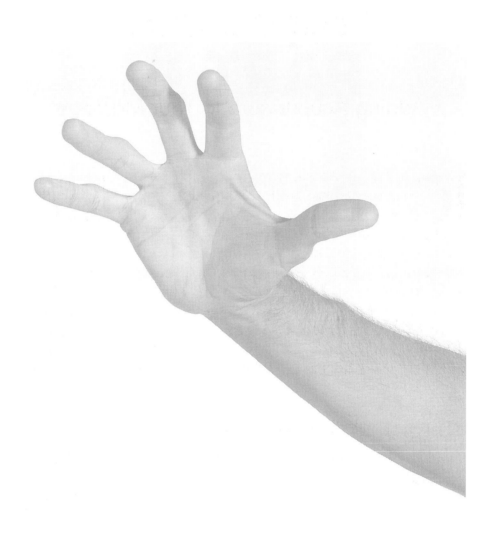

# 13

# Acupressure

## Adding Acupressure to Your Massage

In the hands of a doctor trained in Eastern medicine, acupressure can heal an injured patient. In the hands of a skilled martial artist, it can destroy an opponent.[1] In your hands, it can supercharge your massage.

This chapter will show you how acupressure can make your massage more effective, helping you to feel and perform better. You'll learn why acupressure has been used in Asia for thousands of years, why it's used today by millions of people all over the world, and how it works according to Eastern and Western medicine. You'll learn how to locate and press acupoints to send your Qi, life force, and endorphin energy to every living part of you.

## History of Acupressure

Acupressure is a specialized form of massage that evolved slowly over thousands of years. It's part of a complete healing system used in China and throughout Asia. Acupressure grew out of massage and into acupuncture.

It's easy to see how acupressure would evolve slowly from massage. Over thousands of years, generation after generation of Chinese healers observed how the human body responded to massage. Through trial and error, they discovered points, called acupoints, on the body that were particularly sensitive to touch. When *poked* or *pressed*, these acupoints eliminated pain and improved health.

Chinese physicians observed how pressing acupoints affected not only the specific area touched, but other areas both near and far from the point, concluding that acupoints were connected through a system of internal paths or meridians. They theorized that through these paths flowed a person's life force, or Qi (pronounced "chee" and also spelled chi).[2] Chinese doctors believed that by pressing a patient's acupoints, the patient's life force could be channeled to reduce pain and restore and maintain good health. Over time, Chinese physicians learned to manipulate these acupoints to help the body heal and prevent illness. At first, acupoints were pushed by fingers, but eventually Chinese doctors found more precise ways of stimulating them with pointed sticks and eventually needles.

## Eastern vs. Western Medicine

Centered on radically different philosophies and histories, Eastern and Western medicines are as different as night and day, man and woman, yin and yang. Eastern medicine is based on observing human behavior over thousands of years. Western medicine is based on the latest advances in science and technology. Western medicine's understanding of the human body comes from cutting it open and studying it from the inside out. Eastern medicine's understanding of the human body comes from observing it from the outside and imagining what goes on inside.

In the last thirty years, Western science has come to accept Eastern medicine, specifically acumedicine. Using clinical trials, Western science has found that acupressure relieves pain and can be used to effectively treat illnesses and injuries. Acumedicine has come to be widely used by veterinarians as well. While accepting that acumedicine works, Western science has never accepted Eastern medicine's theories as to why it works.

## TCM and the Life Force

These theories originated with traditional Chinese medicine (TCM). Adherents to TCM believe that your health depends on the flow of energy, or life force, through your body.[3] According to TCM, your body has twelve paths or meridians through which your life force flows.[4] Acupoints are those points on the paths where your life force surfaces and can be manipulated by applying pressure.[5] According to TCM, acupoints can be pressed to slow your life force when it's moving too fast or to speed its flow when it's moving too slowly. Stimulating the life force in this way is believed to prevent illness, restore health, and create a calm energy in the body.[6]

TCM doctors believe that stimulating an acupoint can manipulate life force at three locations:

1. The site of the stimulation;
2. A site along a pathway at a distance from the stimulation;
3. Sites all over the body along pathways all over the body.

Thus, according to TCM, pressing an acupoint may affect you (1) at the muscle pressed; (2) at the surrounding muscles, tissues, joints, and organs; and (3) at muscles in another part of your body.[7] For example, a point in the immediate area of the hip may be used to heal a painful hip muscle. If the acupoint is a particularly powerful one, it can affect your entire body.

TCM identified 360 traditional acupoints. Modern Eastern medicine has identified more than 2,000 acupoints, only 200 of which are regularly used today.[8] Acupoints can be manipulated by needles, fingertips, suction, heat, electricity, lasers, and many massage tools.

## Acupressure Compared to Acupuncture

Westerners sometimes confuse acupressure and acupuncture. Because they're very similar, it's likely that acupuncture evolved from acupressure. Both use the same acupoints to control the same life force through the same paths. The main difference between the two is that acupuncture uses needles and acupressure doesn't. Acupuncture is practiced by physicians and is the more powerful of the two techniques. Acupressure has been used as a method of self-care by athletes and non-athletes since ancient times. For our purposes, acupressure is preferred because it is safer, noninvasive, and you don't have to go to medical school to learn it.

## The Endorphin Force

As of this writing, Western science has not advanced a theory that successfully explains how acumedicine works to treat and prevent illness. Western science has, however, advanced a theory that explains how pressing acupoints reduces pain and produces pleasure. And that may be all you need to know. For it's that pain-reduction, pleasure-enhancing system that you will use to speed your recovery and help you feel better fast.

Advances in Western science's understanding of acumedicine

have dramatically increased acumedicine's use to treat pain in the United States. These advances have taken place in the last thirty years. It is estimated that of the more than one million practitioners outside China who administer acupuncture treatment for pain, more than 300,000 are physicians.[9] Controlled clinical trials show that acupuncture helps from 55 to 85 percent of patients suffering from chronic pain,[10] and in many cases, is even more effective than morphine, which is only effective 70 percent[11] of the time. Additionally, acumedicine does not have the harmful side effects of morphine and other potent pharmaceuticals.

Western science has developed a compelling theory involving endorphins to explain precisely how pressing acupoints relieves pain. Bruce Pomeranz, M.D., Ph.D., is the physician and scientist most responsible for the endorphin response theory. For the last twenty years, he's studied and written extensively on the subject. His research has lead to the discovery of the neural mechanism that acupuncture uses. Dr. Pomeranz has shown that pressing acupoints stimulates the thin nerves in muscles which transmit impulses to your spinal cord. From your spinal cord, the impulses are directed to three centers in your body,[12] which are located in your spinal cord, midbrain, and hypothalamus-pituitary.[13] When stimulated, all three release endorphins and other neurotransmitters.[14] The release of endorphins blocks pain and induces pleasure.

Acupressure mobilizes all three families of endorphins: β-endorphin, enkephalin, and dynorphin.[15] This three-tiered system of pain relief helps you in three ways. When you press an acupoint, three types of endorphins are released by three different neural mechanisms in three different places. First, you get an endorphin release in the area directly surrounding the acupoint you pressed. Second, you may feel the effects of endorphins released at a site along a neuron pathway some distance from the point you pressed. Third, endorphins are released to block pain all over your body, and give you an overall sense of well-being and pleasure. Coolest of all, Western science has shown that the endorphin mechanism acupressure uses is probably the same one that's triggered by endurance running to reduce pain and induce pleasure.[16]

## East Meets West

Although Eastern and Western medicine agree that stimulating acupoints relieves pain and evokes pleasure, they use very different theories to explain why. One uses life force, the other uses endorphin force to explain the powerful effects of acupressure. Whether you believe in the life force or the endorphin force, or see no difference between the two, is up to you. It is reassuring to know that these two great traditions of medicine, one looking from within, the other from without, arrived at the same conclusion: that pressing acupoints can relieve your pain and make you feel better.

## Pressing It

With over 2,000 acupoints in your body, you don't have to know where any of them are to benefit from acupressure. They are everywhere. Just by practicing self-massage, you're bound to activate acupoints. If, however, you want to make your massage more effective, learning where your most potent acupoints are likely to live and how best to press them won't hurt.

If you intend to use acupressure, the first thing you should know is how to press an acupoint. You can use thumbs, fingers, knuckles, elbows, or other massage tools. When first learning, it's best to use either your index or middle finger. For areas of your body that you can't reach, like your back, use one of the massage tools described in Chapter 16.

Try this experiment using a single finger *press* stroke. Place your finger in the depression between your eyebrows. This point is known by acupuncturists as Ex-HN3. Holding your finger at a 90-degree angle to the bridge of your nose, apply a steady gradual pressure.[17] You should feel a pulsing sensation under your finger. This acupoint has a very strong pulse. Most acupoints have a much weaker pulse.[18] Release your finger pressure gradually.

There is no definitive rule for how long to apply pressure. Recommendations vary from five seconds to two minutes. *Press* the point as long as you feel there's a benefit, usually a cessation of sensation. The more you concentrate on the area you're *pressing*, the more effective your *press*.

To get the most out of *pressing* an acupoint, relax your entire body. Focus your attention on the point you're *pressing*. Direct calm, relaxed energy to it. Breathe slowly and deeply into your abdomen, expanding it as you inhale and contracting it as you exhale. Deep breathing improves oxygen intake, improves circulation of blood and energy, and reduces stress. Visualize your intended result. If you're trying to relieve soreness in a muscle, visualize the soreness disappearing. If you're trying to relieve tightness in a muscle, visualize the tightness disappearing.

## How to Find Your Acupoints

Now that you know how to *press* them, let's try to find them. Locating acupoints is more art than science. Like digging for gold, not every place you dig is going to pay off, but every time you do hit one, you'll feel better.

Acupoints usually live in dents in bones, joints, and muscles.[19] Feel for slight indentations. These might be felt as slight depressions in the bone, small spaces between muscle fibers, and slight openings between tendons and muscles.[20] Acupoints range in size from a pinhead to a dime.[21]

You can tell if an acupoint needs to be activated by noticing how sensitive it is to pressure. When massaging your muscles, stop when you hit a tender spot and *press* it to determine whether it's an acupoint. Your ability to find acupoints will improve with time, if you choose to develop it.

If you're new to acupressure, it's impossible to know what an acupoint actually feels like. When you hit one, you may feel a range of sensations which include:

- a dull ache
- a tenderness
- an electrical tingling
- a heaviness
- a warmth

Or you may feel nothing at all. What makes finding acupoints even more challenging is that different acupoints produce different sensations, and the same acupoint may produce different sensations at different times. That's because your body is continually changing. Most of us don't realize it, but we're far more fluid than solid, more space than matter, and more imagination than reality.

## Trying It

First identify a muscle or joint that needs attention. Then, looking at the *Acupoint Body Maps: 25 Power Points for Athletes* at the end of this chapter, locate the acupoint most likely to help based on proximity and description. Apply a *press* or slight *press & roll* stroke. Hold about 30 seconds or until your acupoint is no longer sensitive. You may want to *press* with more than one finger to improve the odds of getting the point.

Finding the acupoint you're looking for is often challenging, but the search may be as important as the discovery. Though you may not find the acupoint you're seeking, your body will benefit from your *pressing*, probing, and exploring. One way to always find the acupoint you're after is to have it indelibly memorialized by your local acupuncturist/tattoo artist. A pen on skin, while less enduring, will work as well if you take a photo of the point for future reference. You may also want to look at an illustrated book of acupoints, such as *The Seirin Pictorial Atlas of Acupuncture*.

The acupoint body maps at the end of this chapter identify twenty-five of the most effective acupoints for athletes. A complete catalogue of all the acupoints in the human body is probably more than you want or need. For more complete guides to acupressure see *Acupressure's Potent Points: A Guide to Self Care for Common Ailments* by Michael Reed Gach and *Essential Anatomy* by Marc Tedeschi. To further deepen your acupressure acumen, consult an accredited acupuncturist.

## In Summary

Whether you live in Beijing or Biloxi, acupressure can be part of every massage you do. Just by practicing massage, you'll activate some of the 2,000 acupoints that live inside you. By following the guidelines in this chapter, you'll be able to improve the quality of your massages by intentionally activating acupoints.

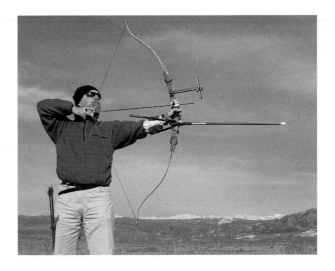

# Acupoint Body Maps:

**GV 14 or Du 14 Water Ditch**
- Restores Calm Energy
- Below big bump on spinal cord between neck and back

**LI 15 Shoulder Bone**
- Improves Shoulder Mobility and Relieves Shoulder Pain
- Outside shoulder, at shoulder bone, feel for indentation in shoulder when arm is held at a right angle to the body

**LI 11 Pool at the Creek**
- Reduces Elbow and Lower Arm Pain
- Bend elbow, acupoint is on outside between bone and crease

**Bl 23 Kidney Shu**
- Relieves Lower Back Pain
- 1.5 thumb widths from spinal cord, in line with navel

**Bl 25 Large Intestine Shu**
- Improves Energy, Reduces Pain
- 1.5 thumb widths from spinal cord, 2 thumb widths below Bl 23

**Ki 6 Shining Sea**
- Increases Running Speed, Relieves Heel and Ankle Pain
- In depression at bottom center of inner ankle knob

**GB 20 Wind Pool**
- Relieves Pain and Relaxes Neck
- In depression behind bony bumps behind ear lobes

**GB 21 Shoulder Well***
- Relaxes Shoulder, Alleviates Pain
- About 2 inches from side of lower neck, in line with GV 14 at the highest point on the shoulder

**GV 4 or Du 4 Gate of Life***
- Improves Sex Drive
- On spinal column in line with navel

**LI 4 Joining Valley***
- Relieves Upper Body Pain, Especially Headaches
- Between thumb and forefinger on back of hand

**GB 30 Jumping Circle**
- Restores Hip Mobility, Relieves Hip Pain, Improves Running Speed
- Outside center of buttocks

**Bl 57 Support the Mountain**
- Relieves Cramps in Calf
- Inside bottom of calf muscle

*Use caution if pregnant

# 25 Power Points for Athletes**

**BI 2 Gathered Bamboo**
- Improves Vision, Relieves Headaches
- Depression under eyebrows next to nose

**GV 26 or DU 26 Water Ditch**
- Opens Senses and Clears Brain
- Half thumb width below nose, between nostrils

**CV 6 or Ren 6 Sea of Energy***
- Strengthen Immune System
- 2 thumb widths below navel

**TW 4 or SJ 4 Active Pond**
- Relieves Wrist, Shoulder, and Back Pain
- Back of wrist, on crease, in line between pinky and ring finger

**Ki 3 Supreme Stream**
- Increases Running Speed, Relieves Ankle and Foot Pain and Swelling
- Between ankle knob and Achilles Tendon

**Sp 4 Grandfather Grandson**
- Relieves Cramps in Arch of Foot
- Side of foot at interior arch, 4 thumb widths from ball of foot

**Lv 3 Great Rushing**
- Relieves Cramps
- Top of foot, 1 to 2 inches back, between big toe and second toe where bones merge

**Ex-HN 3 Hall of Impression**
- Improves Vision
- At indentation between eyebrows

**St 2 Four Whites**
- Relaxes Face
- Directly below pupils, in depression, 1 thumb width below eye sockets

**CV 4 or Ren 4 Gate of Origin***
- Improves Strength and Health
- 3 thumb widths below navel

**St 35 Calf's Nose**
- Relieves Leg Pain
- Bottom exterior of knee cap, feel indentation

**GB 34 Sunny Side of the Mountain**
- Relieves All Muscle and Tendon Issues
- Side of leg, between and behind St 35 and St 36

**St 36 Three Mile Point**
- Strengthens and Energizes Whole Body, Especially Knee
- 3 thumb widths below St 35, 1 thumb width from shinbone
- Some experts believe this is the most important acupoint for athletes

**These are among the most effective acupoints for athletes. Names and numbering system are from Traditional Chinese Medicine.

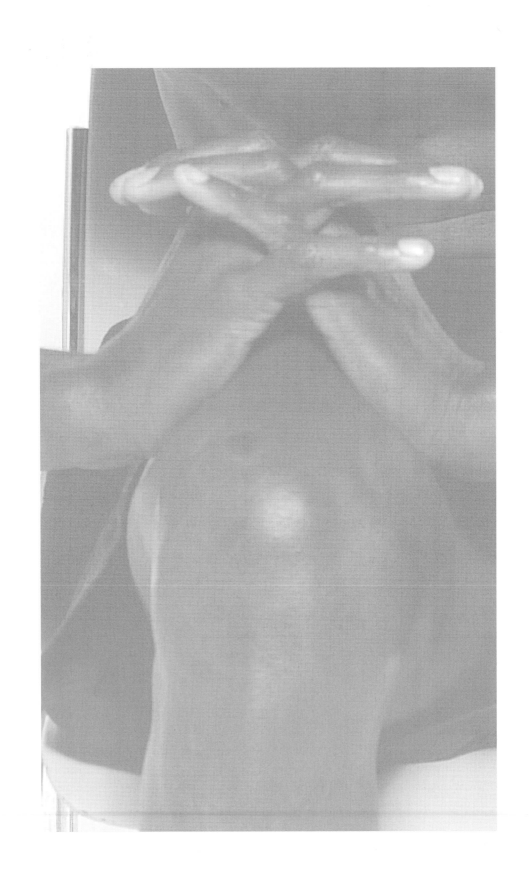

# 14

# Trigger Points

Releasing Knots of Tension
in Your Muscle Fibers

Y ou're bound to trigger them during a massage. You may hit them by accident, by intent, or by divine will. So you should know what trigger points are and how they work. Even if you don't want to trigger them, you should read this chapter so you'll understand why the tiny bursts of pain you feel during a massage may be a good thing.

## What Are Trigger Points?

Trigger points are tiny knots that often form in your muscles.[1] They have the power to reduce your range of motion and damage your athletic performance. When performed correctly, pressing the trigger on a trigger point restores your range of motion and physical performance. Trigger points in muscle fiber are like slip-knots in rope—when touched just right, they disappear.

Trigger points may form in your muscles for many reasons: as the result of improper body mechanics, muscle injuries or strains, physical or mental stress, falls, overuse, or just plain bad luck.[2] They can form when you twist a muscle during a workout or during a hard night's sleep.

At the micro level, trigger points are muscle fibers that have gotten tangled into hard knots.[3] When your muscle fibers over-stretch, they tear. When the muscle fibers heal, they sometimes contract and twist themselves into knots. The knotted muscle fiber reduces your muscle's range of motion and its ability to lengthen. More importantly, the knots block circulation, reducing the flow of nutrient-rich blood to your muscle and the elimination of waste products from your muscle.[4]

## Symptoms

One trouble with trigger points is that their symptoms are often unclear. While pain, inflexible muscles, and stiff joints are often symptomatic of trigger points, sometimes trigger points are not painful. In fact, most athletes suffer these knotted muscle fibers without knowing it. If not triggered, trigger points can last the rest of your life,[5] restricting your range of motion by affecting the muscle and surrounding joint. Trigger points can occur in any muscle in your body, causing localized and referred pain. They very often form at acupoints.

## Identifying Trigger Points

Unless you've experienced their release in the past, you're probably unaware of the benefits of releasing trigger points now. Most athletes find their trigger points by accident, serendipitously. If, during your massage, you find an area in a muscle that is extremely tender, it may be a trigger point. You'll know it's a trigger point if when you apply moderate pressure, it emits a burst of pain.[6] Simply put, a trigger point is the place on a muscle that hurts the most when you press it.

Because they're tangled knots of muscle fiber, trigger points are hard to the touch. If the point has formed in a muscle near your skin, you may feel its hardness when you press it with your finger. In small muscles, the hard area ranges in size from a pin-head to a pea.[7] In large muscles, the area can be as big as a dime.[8]

## Releasing a Trigger Point

Because trigger points rarely form near the skin, it is unlikely that you will be able to feel even large ones with your fingers. The best way to find them is by the pain they emit when you press them. Trigger points almost always cause pain when pressure is directly applied.[9] Paradoxically, triggering one causes and releases pain. When you trigger a trigger point by applying pressure, you feel a burst of pain which fades and then disappears as your muscle fibers stretch, straighten, and unknot. Circulation to the trigger point increases, and the trigger point vanishes. All this relief comes at a price. That price is pain, which lasts anywhere from a few seconds to a minute, the time it takes to straighten your muscle fiber. As the pain increases, your body releases endorphins to reduce pain. You'll feel a tremendous sense of release after a trigger point is fully triggered.

Here's how to deactivate a suspected trigger point. Press directly on the trigger point using your finger or a massage tool. Your finger or massage tool should be perpendicular to your skin and pressed directly on the trigger point.[10] Vary the pressure, increasing and decreasing it until the pain subsides. Slightly vary the angle of pressure. Apply this approach for no more than a minute.[11]

## Hiring a Pro

If you suspect trigger points are causing you pain or limiting your range of motion and you are unable to release them, get professional help. Hire a skilled massage therapist, physical therapist, or acupuncturist. Ask the therapist to teach you how to deactivate your trigger points. If you want to learn more about these points, *The Trigger Point Therapy Workbook* by Clair Davies is a valuable resource.

## In Summary

Trigger points can form in any muscle in your body and last a lifetime. They reduce range of motion, cause pain, and impair muscle performance. By applying pressure to a trigger point, you can make it disappear and improve your physical performance.

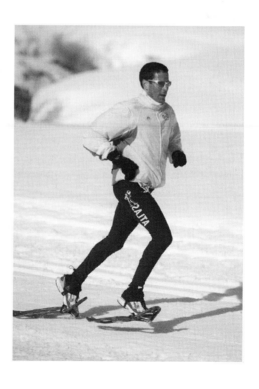

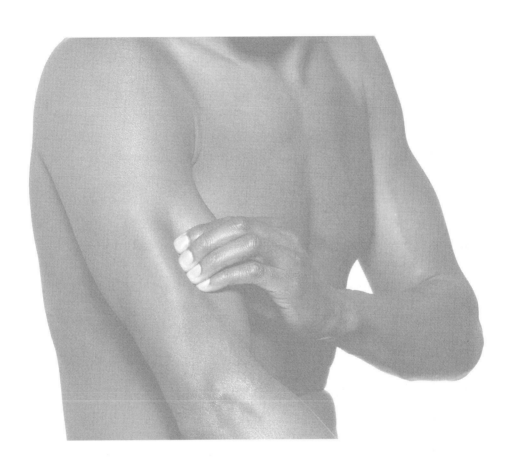

# 15

# Shower Massage

## How to Turn Your Bathroom into a Spa

*"Often one goes for one thing and finds another."*
—Neem Karoli Baba

When you think about it, everything you do in your bathroom is a form of self-massage.

Whether intentionally or unintentionally, effectively or ineffectively, everyone uses self-massage in their bathroom. The purpose of this chapter is to help you learn to use self-massage effectively with intent.

## Your Massage Room

By simply changing your intent, you can make your bathroom massage more effective. All you need to do is change your focus. Then with a little imagination you can turn your bathroom into a spa.

First recognize that every solo activity done in your bathroom is self-massage by another name. Washing, shampooing, conditioning, and combing are all forms of self-massaging. Rubbing, scrubbing, and tubbing are self-massage by other names, as is applying lotions, potions, and ointments. Yes, even brushing your teeth is self-massage! But because most people don't intend them as massage, their full effect is unrealized. By intentionally focusing on these activities as massage, they may become your most effective and, possibly, most joyful massage.

# Conversion

Converting your bathroom into your own personal massage room, a hydrotherapy center for your body, is fast, easy, and free. You don't have to change much of anything except your perspective. Like squinting to see another reality in an Escher print, your bathroom becomes a massage center simply by treating each activity performed in your bathroom as a form of self-massage. Once you see your bathroom as a massage room, you can enjoy the powerful benefits of massage every time you use it.

# Massage Tools

Look carefully and you'll see that your bathroom is loaded with precision instruments for self-massage. Your toothbrush is an ingenious tool designed not only to clean your teeth, but to massage everything that lives in your mouth—your teeth, your gums, and your tongue. While your towel dries you, when used with intent, it can also give you a great massage. In addition to getting you clean, soap and shampoo can give you a soothing massage. Body, hand, and suntan lotions are all slick massage tools. Is there anything in your bathroom that's not used for massage? Dental floss? Q-tips? Razors? Gels? Washcloths? Oils? Mouthwash? Sponges? Luffas? Brushes? Even toilet paper? They're all massage tools.

The wettest and most flexible massage tool in your bathroom is, of course, water. In all its forms, water is a magical tool, a cleansing, healing, life-affirming, massaging force. Flowing from your faucet, a stream of it moistens and massages your hands. In your bath, it surrounds your body, warming, cooling, soothing, and invigorating you. Dancing from your shower, water makes a spectacularly striking massage tool. With the right head, your shower can produce a lively hydromassage anywhere on your beautiful body. Vary the intensity, temperature, and directions of the water and your body will be grateful all day long.

# In the Shower

As an athlete, you probably take more showers than most people. Therefore, you have more to gain by getting a massage every time you shower. You can do that by simply combining massaging with cleaning. Here's how to perform a shower massage that'll make you feel better than clean.

Take off your clothes and get in the shower. Once you've turned on the water, turn off the language center in your brain and focus on your massage. Place your full attention on the exact place the water is hitting your skin. While slowly moving your body to get every part of you wet, keep focused on the water whacking you, massaging you, *pressing* your skin with thousands of tiny drops. Feel it touch different parts of your being as you slowly move, stretch, and twist while adjusting your body's position and water temperature.

## Applying Body Wash

Cleaning your body is a great way to massage your body. Use your hands to glide a body gel or liquid soap directly onto your skin. Bar soap won't do. Gel or liquid soap lets your hands massage your skin. Your hands will usually give you a more effective massage than a block of soap.

To massage the fluid into your skin, begin with your neck, and work your way down, *gliding* your hands over your entire body. Use light strokes to apply the liquid soap, cleaning and massaging as you go. The important thing is to focus your complete attention on what you're feeling and let your body guide your hands, lingering to address sore, tired muscles as needed. Use the full panoply of massage strokes you learned in Chapter 8 to get yourself clean. Breathe deeply into your abdomen as you pay special attention to those parts of your body that seem sore or tight from your last workout. Use gentle cat-like stretches to stretch and relax your muscles as you massage your skin clean.

## Facial Massage

Massaging your face clean requires your full attention. Start by gliding the gel onto your skin. Then *press & roll* it in with your fingertips. Shift your attention between feeling the water massaging you and feeling your hands massaging you. Direct your awareness to one, and then to the other. Then lightly *drum* your face awake with your fingertips. Voila, the perfect clean for the perfect face. You can apply this technique to massaging your whole body clean.

## Shampoo and Condition

Shampooing should be an arousing massage for your scalp. Conditioning is a second chance to arouse your follicles. Both bring fresh rich blood to the part of you that lives between your ears.

Use your fingers to *press & roll* shampoo and conditioner onto your scalp. Massage your entire head with a series of *press & roll* strokes. Continue to keep the language center in your brain off.

## Shaving in the Shower

Shaving can be more than a way to remove unwanted hair. Turn shaving into self-massage by turning your full attention to feeling the blade *glide* against your skin. Pay close attention because the razor can be a dangerous massage tool.

## Handheld Showerhead

A handheld showerhead is a powerful massage tool. It allows you to vary the intensity, angle, and pulsation pattern of your shower massage. With it you can massage hard to reach parts of your body with invigorating blasts of water. Hold the showerhead inches from your head or inches from the bottom of your foot, directing the flow of water to the exact spot on your anatomy that most needs it. A handheld showerhead adds power to your shower.[1]

## Water Temperature

By changing the water temperature, you change the effect of your shower massage. Heat is wonderful therapy for sore muscles. It increases circulation and warms your muscles, making them more flexible. Cold water wakes you up and invigorates you but may cause shrinkage.[2]

## The Bath and Beyond

Although it may not seem so at first, relaxing in your bathtub is an excellent way to get a massage. The water pressure presses against your whole being, compressing your muscles, heating or cooling you, relaxing or stimulating you. Use your hands to *glide*, *squeeze*, *squeeze & roll*, *press*, *press & roll*, and *drum* yourself clean. These strokes are especially effective under water.

A warm bath can be a totally relaxing massage. Add Jacuzzi jets and you can relax every muscle in your body. Beyond the bath, using the heat in steam rooms and saunas can help you massage more deeply into muscles.

Ice can be nice. Dunk your body in a body of cold water and feel the instant effects of an invigorating ice-cold massage. Apply massage strokes as needed, and your body will feel the benefits all day. A cold-water massage is one of the best ways to recover from a tough workout or competition. A cold lake, stream, ocean, or bathtub works wonders.

# After the Shower

## Hand Drying

A terrific shower massage doesn't have to end with the shower. If you do it right, drying is an invigorating massage as well. Gliding your hands over your moist skin is a slick way to dry off. Try shaking off any excess water with a little *rock & roll* stroke. Most canines have mastered this stroke. You can too. It's a drying and stimulating stroke. You'll feel energy pumping through your entire moist being.

## Washcloth Drying

To get fully dry you'll need a towel. Using a large towel to dry your skin can give you a nice rub. But for a great massage, try a washcloth or small towel. Using a washcloth to massage your entire body dry may seem goofy, but it forces you to pay attention to the massage part of drying. Use light *squeezing* strokes to massage your muscles and dry your skin. *Gliding* the cloth over your body will dry your skin but won't massage your muscles. Try tapping yourself dry, by using a *drumming* stroke on a towel held over your body. It's a great way to dry off and get going.

## Drying Hair and Massaging Scalp

Drying your hair can produce another rewarding scalp massage. To massage your scalp while drying your hair, just place a small towel between your hair and your fingers and use your fingers to *press & roll* your scalp while the towel absorbs water from your hair.

## Body Lotions, Oils, and Creams

Massaging body lotions into your skin with a firm *gliding* stroke gives you a moist massage. Applying facial lotions using a *press & roll* stroke should give your face a lift and a massage.

## Ear Massage

*Squeezing & rolling* while cleaning and drying your ears gives them an invigorating massage. *Gliding* the heels of your hands over your ears, closing your eyes, and listening deeply is a trip.

### Hand Wash

*Gliding* your hands clean while rubbing them against each other is an effective way to massage your hands and reward them for massaging and cleaning the rest of you.

## In Summary

When in the bathroom, focus your attention on your massage. You'll still get cleaned and groomed, but you'll also get massaged, which will make your body happy. And if your body is happy, your heart and mind will follow.

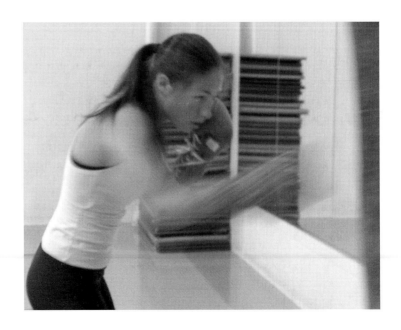

# 16

# Massage Tools

## Simple Tools to Improve
## Your Power and Reach

**M**any are called. Few are chosen. Here are some massage tools that you should choose to improve your massage: Thera Cane®, Body Back Buddy™, Dolphin Massager, Knobble®, Trigger Wheel®, Foam Roller, and The SockBall Self-Massage Tool (homemade). Each tool is designed to make your massage more effective. Each can be used to supplement the massage strokes described in this book. Admittedly, some look like modern versions of medieval torture devices. That's okay. Most athletes know that embedded in therapy and pleasure is a hint of pain.

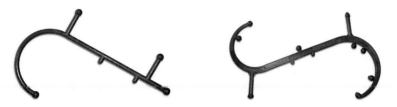

## Thera Cane® and Body Back Buddy™

**Description of Products:** The Thera Cane® and Body Back Buddy™ are two extremely effective general purpose self-massage tools. They do things for you that your hands alone cannot do. The Thera Cane® is made of green fiberglass, shaped like a cane, and sports six knobs. It's about two feet long and fifteen inches wide. The Body Back Buddy™ is made of high-impact-glass-filled nylon polymer, shaped like an "S," and sports eleven knobs, eight rounded and three pointed. It weighs 1.5 pounds, is about two feet long and twenty inches wide.

**How to Use:** Each comes with its own manual describing use.

**Purpose:** Each tool lets you apply pressure to areas that are hard to reach with your hands, like your back. They also let you direct pressure anywhere on your body.

**Effect:** Both the Thera Cane® and the Body Back Buddy™ stimulate acupoints and trigger points, and can give your back a good massage. They can help give you a deeper, more effective overall massage as well.

**Price & Manufacturer:**  About $40. Thera Cane Company. About $40, Body Back Company.

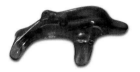

# Dolphin Massager

**Description of Product:** This massage tool, shaped like a dolphin, is less than seven inches long, weighs about six ounces, and is made of hard plastic. The Dolphin Massager comes in a variety of bright colors, and is a surpisingly effective self-massage tool.

**How to Use:** Just glide its belly along your skin or use its fins, tail, or nose to apply pressure wherever your body needs it. The Dolphin comes with its own set of instructions.

**Purpose:** The Dolphin works as an extension of your hands. It lets you add intensity to your stroke and do a few things your hands can't do. It can be used for *gliding, pressing, pressing & rolling,* and, by twisting it, you can get an effective *squeeze & roll* stroke.

**Effect:** The Dolphin Massager intensifies *gliding* and *pressing* strokes. It lets you apply more pressure with less effort. The Dolphin concentrates pressure on acupoints and trigger points. It's been known to stir some endorphin cocktails as well.

**Price & Distributor:** From $12 to $18. Bodycare Companions.

# The Knobble®

**Description of Product:** The Knobble® is an elegant, smooth, hard wood massage tool. It's shaped like a rounded wooden mushroom. It fits comfortably in the palm of your hand, is about two-and-a-quarter-inches long, and weighs about two ounces.

**How to Use:** Place the wide end in the palm of your hand and the narrow end on the area of your body you want to massage. Apply pressure and you've got it. It comes with instructions.

**Purpose:** The Knobble® lets you focus pressure when using compression strokes, such as *presses* and *press & rolls*.

**Effect:** The Knobble® concentrates pressure on acupoints and trigger points. It lets you apply more pressure with less effort. The Knobble® improves the intensity of your massage, giving you a deeper, more effective massage. Releases endorphins.

**Price & Manufacturer:** From $12 to $15. Knobble Associates.

## TriggerWheel®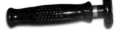

**Description of Product:** The TriggerWheel® is a compact six-inch, six-ounce device. It appears to be little more than a handle with a two-inch wheel attached. However, the TriggerWheel®, made of nylon and steel, is a deceptively simple powerful massage tool.

**How to Use:** Roll the wheel over the part of your body that needs attention.

**Purpose:** To relax tight, tender muscles and encourage good circulation.

**Effect:** Relieves muscle pain and stiffness.

**Price & Manufacturer:** About $20. RPI of Atlanta.

## Foam Roller

**Description of Product:** Foam Rollers are made of hard Styrofoam, and shaped like cylinders. They come in different sizes varying from 12 x 3 inches to 48 x 4 inches (lengths and diameters). Choose one that fits your needs.

**How to Use:** Place the Foam Roller on the floor. Lie, sit, or stand on the Roller and roll it under your body's weight. By pressing your weight against the rounded hard Styrofoam surface, your muscles get a high compression massage.

**Purpose:** Relieves muscle soreness all over your body. Depending on the size you choose, it's particularly good for your upper legs, butt, back, and the bottoms of your feet.

**Effect:** Using your body's weight to roll a muscle over hard Styrofoam relieves muscle tension. Think of it working like a rolling pin smoothing dough. The cylinder rolls under your muscles, aligning muscle fibers, restoring circulation, and relieving muscle soreness. Getting off the roller will feel much better than getting on it.

**Price & Distributor:** From $12 to $26, depending on size. OPTP.

# Sockball Self-Massage Tool

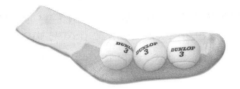

**Description of Product:** The SockBall is a massage tool that you can make yourself. It's three tennis balls and a sock. You can use it to massage your back, your front, and anywhere else that feels good.

**Materials Needed:** You'll need three tennis balls and a sock. The sock should be about eighteen inches long.

**Assembly Instructions:** Put the tennis balls in the sock. Voila, you now have a SockBall Self-Massage Tool.

**Cost:** Three tennis balls and a sock, maybe $3.

**Stroke:** Stand with your back against a blank wall and lean on the balls. Or, while seated in a hard-backed chair, place the SockBall between your back and the chair back.

**Upper Back:** Start with your right side. Dangle the SockBall over your right shoulder, between you and the wall or the chair back. Massage your upper back by leaning against the balls and moving your body from side to side and up and down. Continue to hold the sock over your shoulder. Lower the balls to massage lower parts of your upper back. Repeat the process on your left side.

**Lower Back:** To massage your lower back, slide the balls into the middle of the sock and hold the sock behind you with both hands so that the balls are parallel to the ground. Lean your weight against one or two of the balls, and sway to your left and right. Move your lower back from side to side and up and down. Massage as much of your lower back as you can.

**Glute Massage:** Slide the sock down a little farther to get a great glute massage. Do one side and then the other. Take time to relieve all the tensions that have accumulated in your butt muscles. Experiment with different moves and intensities. A twisting motion is often very effective.

**Upper Leg Massage:** You can use the SockBall to massage your upper legs. Lean sideways with the SockBall between you and the wall. The balls should be parallel to the floor. Use an up-and-down or back-and-forth motion to massage the side of your thigh. Massage the front of your thighs (quadriceps) using the same technique.

**Intensity:** The more weight you place against the balls, the more intense your massage. With practice, you'll be able to give yourself a great back massage using the SockBall Self-Massage Tool.

**Note on Use:** You can use the SockBall on the floor just like a Foam Roller. It's great for massaging the bottoms of your feet.

## In Summary

Massage tools can make your massage more effective and pleasurable. Try the Thera Cane®, Body Back Buddy,™ Dolphin Massager, Knobble®, Trigger Wheel®, Foam Roller and SockBall Massage Tool. You'll like them.

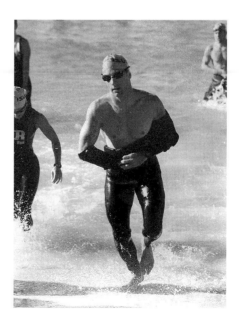

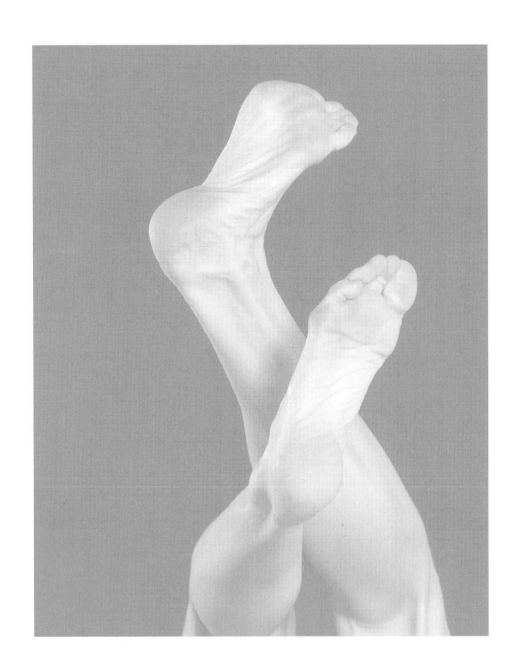

# 17

# Feeling Even Better

Using Power Breathing, Visualization, and Meditation to Enrich Your Massage

*Power breathing*, visualization, and meditation are three ways to increase the quality of your massage. All three will improve the effectiveness and pleasure you get from self-massage. In turn, increased effectiveness will improve your athletic performance. Here's a short description of how each one works and how they'll improve your massage.

## Power Breathing

While breathing is not optional, the way you breathe is. By practicing power breathing during self-massage, you can improve your mood, energy, and the quality of your massage. The *power* in power breathing does not refer to the intensity with which you breathe but the powerful effect it has. Think of power breathing as breathing with intent. It's really just paying attention to your breath so that you can control it to meet your needs. Athletes do this all the time. Every sport has its own breathing pattern associated with it.

Medical scientists say that breathing is the only biological function that can be completely voluntary or completely involuntary. Involuntary breathing is what most of us do most of the time to stay alive. A few athletes who have learned to pay attention to their breath have gotten extraordinary results. By paying attention to their breath, yogis have learned to control their body temperature, heart rate, and can go for days without breathing.[1] But you don't have to give up breathing for even a minute to get the benefits of power breathing. All you have to do is pay attention to your breath long enough to control it.

### Mood

Changing your breathing pattern during self-massage can improve your mood. All athletes experience a change in mood every time they work out. Part of that mood change is the result of a changed breathing pattern. You can change your mood during self-massage in much the same way, just by focusing on your breath and changing its depth, cadence, intensity, or even its place of intake.

### Energy

Changing your breathing pattern during self-massage will also affect your energy level. Here's why: we use oxygen to burn fuel in our bodies. This creates the energy that powers us. If you want to burn fuel faster to create more energy, you have to take in more oxygen. To accomplish that, all you have to do is breathe more intensely. It works every time. As a general rule, breathing harder produces more energy, breathing softer is relaxing.

### Breathing during Massage

The breathing pattern you adopt during each massage should reflect your goal for that particular massage. For instance, deep breathing through your mouth energizes you,[2] while slow, easy breathing through your nose relaxes you. In either case, use your abdomen to control your breath while practicing self-massage. (When you inhale, your lower back comes in; when you exhale your belly button comes in.) While practicing self-massage, be aware of your breathing. Experiment with different power breathing patterns, cadence, intensity, and nose breathing to improve your mood and energy level.

# Visualization

Visualization can also improve your massage. An integral part of most native and world religions, it has been used for thousands of years to elevate experience and performance.[3] The world's best athletes use visualization techniques to increase performance.[4] They know from experience that visualization works.

Visualization lets athletes preview an event before they perform it, allowing them to affect the outcome. When done correctly, visualization increases performance because it prepares athletes before they compete. As it allows them to see and feel themselves having the experience before they actually have it, visualization lets athletes become more fully absorbed in their actual competition.

Similarly, you can use visualization to enhance your massage experience. The more intensely you devote your attention to an activity, the more you'll enjoy it and the better you'll perform. Here are some visualization sets that will increase the effectiveness of your massage:

### Learning Self-Massage Set

To start with, visualize yourself learning massage. See how simple and easy it is to learn. Visualize how powerful it will make you feel every time you use it. Visualize how much pleasure you'll feel to relieve your muscle pain whenever you want. See yourself feeling better anytime you want. Visualize yourself enjoying improved athletic performance and health.

### Before Starting a Self-Massage Set

Before you begin a massage, visualize yourself enjoying the massage. Don't be afraid to exaggerate when using visualization. Visualize muscle pain evaporating like sweat on a hot day. Visualize every corpuscle of your being pulsing with pleasure. Visualize the massage filling you with energy. Do this before every massage and you'll feel a new sense of power every time you finish your massage.

### During Self-Massage Set

Use visualization during your massage to see inside your body. Picture fresh, healthy blood loaded with pure oxygen and vital nutrients flooding your muscles. See polluted wastes forced out of your muscles with each stroke. See energy flowing through you. Picture mechanical energy leaving your hands and reforming into heat energy on your skin, and electrochemical energy throughout your body. See your body filled with this new energy. You may want to picture it as lightning bolts or high-octane juices. Visualize your muscle fibers being stretched apart and regaining their flexibility. Visualize muscle pain melting away, like snow on a hot day. Visualize tiny endorphin cocktails emptying into your system and nourishing you. Visualize your muscles healing, getting stronger, and expanding to Hulk-like proportions.

Experiment and have fun with your visualizations. Use whatever visualization techniques make you feel good.

## Meditation: Silence of the Mind

All great athletes know that to perform best they must be fully absorbed in what they're doing. To get the greatest benefit from self-massage, you must be fully absorbed in it. Your focus, attention, and concentration should be on your massage. Turn off the language center in your brain and let your body do your thinking for you. When you become fully absorbed in your massage, you'll find your body directing your hands. Your massage will be performed spontaneously and intuitively without your conscious effort.

## In Summary

You'll get a more effective massage if you use power breathing, visualization, and meditation. These techniques may also be used to improve athletic performance during training and competition.

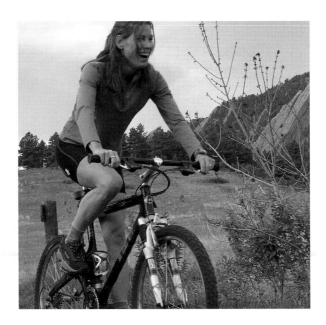

# 18

# When Not to Self-Massage

## When to Refrain from Self-Massage and Consult a Medical Professional

This chapter addresses four different but related questions:

1. Are there times when you should not use self-massage?

2. Should you use self-massage if you have significant health problems?

3. Should you treat serious injuries with self-massage?

4. When should you hire a massage therapist?

## Contraindications for Massage

There are times when even the best activities should be forgone. Contraindications for self-massage include:

| | |
|---|---|
| Artificial blood vessels | Lumps |
| Bleeding | Muscle ruptures |
| Blood clots | Open wounds |
| Broken bones | Pacemakers |
| Burns | Phlebitis |
| Bursitis | Rheumatoid arthritis |
| Contusions | Skin infections |
| Fevers | Sores |
| Gout | Tendon ruptures |
| Heart transplants | Thrombosis |
| Infections | Tumors |

# Illness & Health Problems

If you have a serious illness or health issue, you should consult a professional healthcare provider before starting a self-massage or an exercise program.

## Pregnancy

Self-massage can be a pleasant gift when you're pregnant. Always be gentle with yourself. Never do deep abdominal massage while pregnant. If your pregnancy is complicated by diabetes, hypertension, or any other disorder, you should consult your physician before starting a self-massage or exercise program.

## Treating Injuries

You should not self-treat significant injuries. Seek professional medical care when you're injured. Even if you are a healthcare professional, get a second opinion. Examples of injuries for which you should seek professional health care include the following:

- Sprains
- Torn muscles, ligaments, or cartilage
- Numbness
- Extreme sensitivity to touch
- Severe muscle spasms
- Prolonged or significant swelling
- Large internal scar tissue felt as a hard lump
- All the contraindicators previously identified

# Getting It from a Pro

There are many good reasons to consult a professional massage therapist. Three that leap to mind are injury, injury, and injury. Massage therapists explore soft tissue more knowledgeably than most other healthcare providers. Your body has two types of tissue: hard and soft. Hard is bone. Soft is everything else. Massage therapists work with soft tissue. If the problem is sports related, it makes sense to consult a massage therapist who works with athletes.

Learning self-massage is another good reason to consult a massage therapist. If there's anything in this book that you are unsure about, ask a qualified professional for help. Good massage therapists encourage their patients to use self-massage to complement their therapy. Your massage therapist will probably be happy to help you learn self-massage techniques to improve your health and well being.

Massage therapy and self-massage are not mutually exclusive; in fact, they go hand in hand. Professional massage therapists can reach places that your hands cannot. Their hands may go more deeply into your muscles than yours. Their hands may be able to touch you in ways that yours cannot, and theirs may relax you in ways yours may not.

According to Neal Henderson, MS, CSCS , coordinator of sports science at the Boulder Center for Sports Medicine:

> [S]elf massage can be quite helpful for the athlete to learn how to listen to their body . . . . One of the major disadvantages of self-massage is that not all areas of the body can be appropriately addressed. Another difficultly comes in being able to apply the appropriate force to massage a specific area, while promoting relaxation within the target tissues. On a more frequent basis, self-massage is an excellent tool for use by the athlete. I do believe that less frequent sessions with a professional massage therapist will allow the athlete to gain benefits that are not possible to be reached through self-massage.

Although they have much in common, massage therapy and self-massage are not identical. Neither is better than the other, as they meet similar and different needs. Use each one as you need it. Each is a great way to feel great.

## In Summary

Get help from a professional massage therapist when you need it, especially when you have a serious injury, or health problem. You can learn a lot from a good massage therapist. Find one that you like, who can help you learn, heal, and feel better.

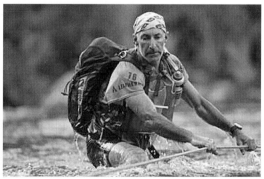

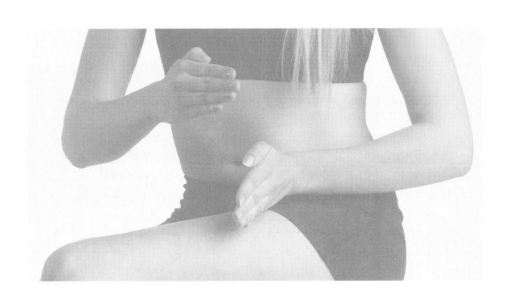

# 19

# Coaches and Personal Trainers

## How to Make Your Whole Team Feel Great

**Skip this chapter if you're not a coach or a personal trainer.**

If you are a coach or a personal trainer, self-massage may be the most effective training tool you can offer your athletes. Whether you work with competitive or noncompetitive athletes, self-massage will improve their athletic performance. Using self-massage will reduce your athletes' rate of injuries, recovery time, and sore muscles. It will increase their self-confidence, morale, overall health, and happiness. But you already know that. The question is how to communicate it to your athletes. You might start with a brief history of massage.

## History

Tell them that "Athletes have been using massage for thousands of years to warm up before competitions and to recover after competitions. Massage was used by athletes in the original Greek Olympic games held in 776 BC. Twenty-seven hundred years later, massage is still used all over the world by elite athletes." That's enough history. The only duty we owe history is to condense it. Move on to the present before they fall asleep.

## The Present

Tell them that "Today, all sports programs should provide athletes with frequent massage. Unfortunately, only the wealthiest teams have the financial resources to do so. With self-massage, every one of you can enjoy the benefits of massage.

"Most of you have too much to do and too little time to do it. Self-massage lets you receive the benefits of massage while doing other things, like studying, attending classes, watching TV, traveling to away games, and waiting. When you're young, you always feel like you're waiting for something to happen. Self-massage will give you something to do while you're waiting."

## Stretching and Massage

Then tell them something about stretching and massage to wake them up, like, "In the Middle Ages, stretching was used as a form of torture. For many of you, stretching is still considered an instrument of pain. But massage is one of the most pleasurable things you can do for your body without breaking the law." Tell them how stretching and massage are "good ways to complete a workout. Both are used to affect circulation and stretch muscles. Self-massage may be combined with an easy stretching routine to make your stretches even more effective."

## Team Benefits

Then tell them what they'll get if they practice self-massage:

- Better warm-ups before workouts
- Improved athletic performance and fitness
- Reduced incidents of injury
- Reduced recovery time between workouts
- Relief from muscle pain and soreness
- Increased range of motion and overall health
- Improved mood, energy, and ability to relax
- Increased self-confidence and body awareness

## Teaching Self-Massage

The easiest way to teach your athletes self-massage is to give them a copy of this book and encourage them to devote ten minutes to self-massage after every workout. Review the basic strokes in Chapter 8 with them. You'll find that your athletes will learn self-massage quickly and use it effectively.

## In Summary

Like the insights into human nature you give your athletes, self-massage is a lifetime benefit and resource for them. Once their season is over, they may not use stretching or most of the drills they've learned, but they will use self-massage.

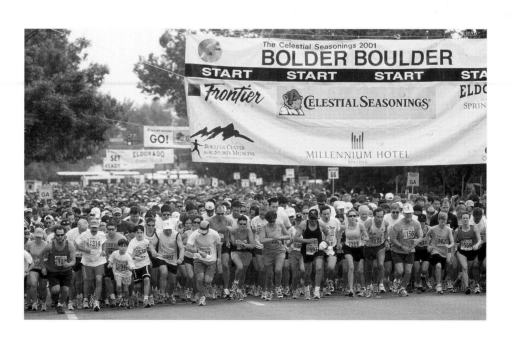

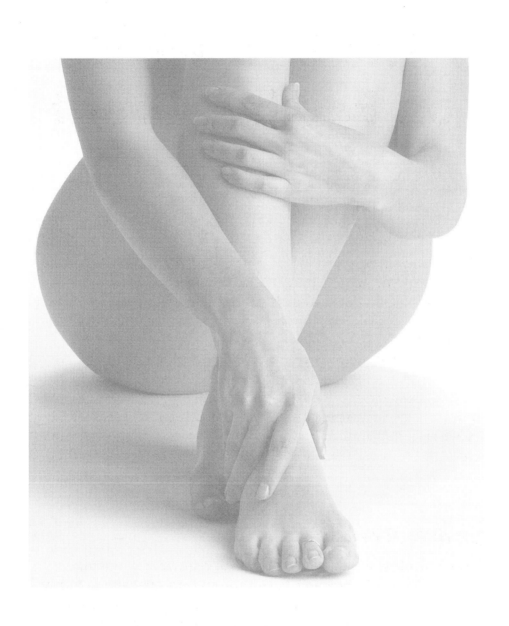

# 20

# The Last Word on Feeling Great

## The Power Is in Your Hands

It's always a good feeling to start the final chapter of a book. It usually means the end is near. But here it means the beginning is near. A new beginning, in which your life as an athlete can be much better because you make self-massage a part of your routine.

For this book to help you become a healthier, happier, and better athlete, you must use the techniques and ideas presented in the last nineteen chapters. Practice massage on a regular basis (at least three times per week but preferably every day) to best experience its benefits. If you put this book down now and never use it again, you'll have gained nothing. If, after finishing this chapter, you adopt a program of regular massage, you'll lift your athletic performance to the next level.

## Sports Benefits

Let's look at what you can expect with regular self-massage. Athletically, you'll experience significant improvement not only in your performance, but in your fitness level and the pleasure you get from sports. Here's why: self-massage works directly on your muscles to relieve soreness, tension, and pain after workouts. By reducing muscle soreness, tension, and pain, you'll recover more quickly after exercise. The quicker you recover, the more effective your training and the better your fitness level, which leads to increased athletic performance.

Self-massage will also reduce your risk of injury. That, in itself, will make your training more effective, because, to improve athletic performance, you have to train consistently. To be consistent, of course, you have to avoid injuries that interfere with your training. By using self-massage, you'll reduce the number of injuries and their severity. Self-massage will help you avoid injury by preparing you for workouts, speeding your recovery between workouts, and helping you focus your attention on the parts of your body that need it.

## General Benefits

In addition to directly improving athletic performance, self-massage will indirectly improve your performance by improving your health and mood.

Over time, your immune system will grow stronger, you'll have fewer and milder illnesses. You'll become more relaxed and more comfortable with yourself as you discover you're less anxious and less affected by the harmful effects of stress.

The ability to relieve pain and make yourself feel good will empower you and carry into everything you do. It's an ability that is entirely self-contained. No pain, all gain.

With regular self-massage, you'll notice an improvement in your mood. You'll feel happier. You'll discover a calm yet increased energy that supports your activities and helps you accomplish your goals on and off the field.

## Self Knowledge

Best of all, by using self-massage, you'll gain a better understanding of yourself. Science has shown, and human experience has proven, that which you devote your attention to thrives. Self-massage focuses your attention on you. If you practice it regularly, you will thrive.

## The Whole Enchilada

In a way, every sport you play, every workout you perform is a form of self-massage. Whether it's running or swimming, biking or basketball, it's all massage. Every athletic move you make, every action you take results in a massage to part of your body.

Walking or running gives your feet a massage. Swimming uses water to massage your entire body. Handball massages your hands. Horseback riding and mountain biking massage your butt. Golf massages your wallet. Yoga massages your insides and your outsides. Skydiving, cycling, surfing, and skiing use rushing air to massage your skin. Contact sports like football, wrestling, boxing, and martial arts are forms of high-impact massage.

In one way or another, every move you make, every step you take is a form of self-massage. Whether it's sports or eating, sex or sleeping—every action you take results in a massage to either your insides or outsides. Every move you make may be your body's attempt to get massaged. Eating and digesting massages your insides. Sex can massage your insides and outsides. When you think about it, sex is little more than a mutual massage done to exhaustion. In this sense, massage may be the real goal of life, and procreation a mere side effect. Life as we know it may be nothing more than our bodies' attempts to get a good massage.

With that in mind, it makes sense to give your body the massage it needs whenever it wants one. Using the techniques presented in this book, you'll be able to fine-tune your massage to do just that.

## In Summary

Self-massage is the power to feel great any time you want. Not an art or a science but a pleasure, regular self-massage will make you a better athlete. It will also make you healthier and happier.

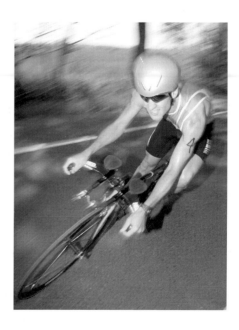

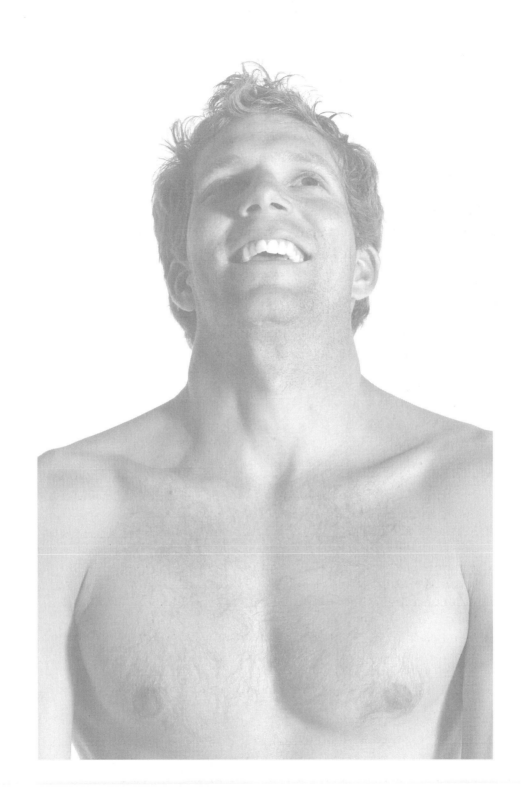

# Notes

## Chapter 1

1. Field, *Touch Therapy*, xii.

## Chapter 2

1. Field, *Touch Therapy*, 35; and Grossberg, "Interaction with Pet Dogs: Effects on Human Cardiovascular Response," 12, 20–27.
2. Field, *Touch Therapy*, 35–41.

## Chapter 3

1. Merriam Webster's Dictionary, on-line edition, http://www.m-w.com/.
2. Braun, *Science of Happiness*, 2.
3. Vickers, *Massage and Aromatherapy*, 92.
4. Field, *Touch Therapy*, 211–214.
5. Ibid., 179–186.
6. Ibid., 205–210.
7. Ibid., 161–165.
8. Ibid., 123–134.
9. Ibid., 99–106.
10. Ibid., 106–111.
11. Field et al. *Adolescence*, 903–911.
12. Shulman and Jones, "The Effectiveness of Massage Therapy on Reducing Anxiety in the Workplace," 160-173.
13. Kubsch, Nuveau, and Vandertie, "Effect of Cutaneous Stimulation on Pain Reduction in Emergency Department Patients," 25–32; and Field, *Touch Therapy*, 45–91.
14. Richards, "The Effect of Back Massage and Relaxation Intervention on Sleep," 288–299.
15. Field et al., "Massage and Relaxation Therapies' Effects on Depressed Adolescent Mothers," 903–911; Leivadi et al., "Therapy and Relaxation Effects on University Dance Students," 108-112.; and Field, *Touch Therapy*, 145–150.
16. Hernandez-Reif, "Premenstrual Syndrome Symptoms Are Relieved by Massage Therapy," 9–15.
17. Field, *Touch Therapy*, 106–115.
18. Hernandez-Reif et al., "Migraine Headaches Are Reduced by Massage Therapy," 1–11.
19. Field et al., "Children with Asthma Have Improved Pulmonary Functions after Massage Therapy," 854–858.
20. Field et al., "Massage Therapy Reduces Anxiety and Enhances EEG Pattern of Alertness and Math Computations," 197–205.
21. Hart, "Anorexia Nervosa Symptoms Are Reduced by Massage Therapy," 289–299.
22. Field, *Touch Therapy*, 201–217.

23. Mayo Clinic, www.mayoclinic.com.
24. Field, *Touch Therapy*, 113.
25. Ibid.
26. Vickers, *Massage and Aromatherapy*, 125.
27. Field, *Touch Therapy*, 45.
28. Ibid., 67 and 134–145.
29. Ibid., 45–52.
30. Ibid., 145–150.
31. Ibid., 23–32.
32. Ibid., 161–165.
33. Stephen Braun describes how drugs are marketed in *The Science of Happiness*, 1–26.
34. Eisenberg et al., "Trends in Alternative Medicine Use in the United States, 1990-1997," 1569–1575.
35. Weil, *Health and Healing*, 96–97.
36. Field, *Touch Therapy*, xii.
37. Ibid., xii and 145–150.

## Chapter 4

1. Field, *Touch*, 76–81.
2. Weil, *Health and Healing*, 61.
3. Field, *Touch Therapy*, 165.

## Chapter 5

1. Calvert, "Pages from History: The Greek Gymnasium," 172–175.
2. Armstrong, *It's Not About the Bike*, 85, 269, 286.
3. Ibid., 229.
4. Johnson, *The Healing Art of Sports Massage*, 152.
5. Shrier, "Stretching Before Exercise Does Not Reduce the Risk of Local Muscle Injury: A Critical Review of the Clinical and Basic Science Literature," 221–227; Shrier, "Myths and Truths of Stretching," 324–325; and Kurz, *Stretching Scientifically*, 11.
6. Smith, "The Effects of Athletic Massage on Delayed Onset Muscle Soreness, Creatine Kinase, and Neutrophil Count: A Preliminary Report," 93–99.
7. Hernandez-Reif, "University Dance Students Show Increased Range of Motion Following Massage Therapy," 183–189. Massage improved range of motion, mood, and performance when dancers received massages twice per week for one month.
8. Vickers, *Massage and Aromatherapy*, 98.
9. Weil, *Health and Healing*, 58.

## Chapter 6

1. Serotonin is produced by the pineal gland in the heart of the brain. It's been referred to as the molecule of happiness. It's a neurotransmitter, which affects mood, sleep, appetite, and other

bodily functions. Low serotonin levels correlate with depression, anxiety, and insomnia. Pharmaceuticals have been developed to increase serotonin levels. The most effective natural way to increase serotonin levels is physical exercise. LSD and serotonin have similar chemical structures; LSD mimics serotonin in the brain.

2. Dopamine is a hormone produced in the hypothalamus. It's been linked to addiction, pleasure, and desire. It is a neurotransmitter which correlates with feelings of satisfaction at the relief of hunger, thirst, and sexual desire. Recent research indicates that dopamine, long thought to mediate pleasure, in fact, mediates desire. Its effect can be mimicked by cocaine and amphetamines. www.heroin.org/dopamine.

3. Anandamide is a chemical produced in the human brain that was discovered in 1992. It means "bliss" in Sanskrit. It's a neurotransmitter whose activity correlates with changes in mood, memory, appetite, and pain. Anandamide's chemical composition is very similar to that of tetrahydrocannabinol (THC), the active ingredient in marijuana. Anandamide breaks down very quickly in the human body so the high it produces is not likely to last long. Chocolate contains substances that resemble anandamide. http://www.runnersworld.com/article/0,5033,s6-197-200-0-1102,00.html, and http://www.healthandfitnessmag.com/OnTheRun apr05.htm.

4. Serotonin, dopamine, anandamide, and endorphins are all produced by the human body. Each one of these has what might be characterized as an evil twin, a chemical compound produced in the lab that chemically looks like one of these natural substances but is slightly different. That difference can be enormously destructive. These destructive drugs—LSD, cocaine, amphetamines, and morphine—fit into the same receptors in the brain as do serotonin, dopamine, anandamide, and endorphins. The human body mistakes the destructive drugs for their natural biochemical twin and the result can be devastating.

5. Kolata, "Runner's High? Endorphins? Fiction, Some Scientists Say," May 21, 2002.

6. Levinthal, *Messengers of Paradise*, 113–116.

7. Ibid., 98–100

8. If you have ever had a near-death experience, the feeling is similar to the one felt during an endorphin peak experience. If you listen to the recorded messages of people on September 11, 2001, trapped at the top of the World Trade Center, who knew death was certain, you get a sense of enormous calm and clarity in their voices and messages. It is speculated that this feeling is not unlike the experience some athletes report during an endorphin-peak experience. Some say the feeling is also similar to that experienced during intense meditation or religious rituals. It is one of being fully alive, sentient, calm, and powerful although death may be imminent.

9. Pelé, *My Life and the Beautiful Game, 51*; and Murphy, *In The Zone*, 94.

## Chapter 7

1. Ylinen, *Sports Massage*, 13.
2. Burke, *Optimal Muscle Performance and Recovery*, 13–14; and Juhan, *Job's Body*, 116–132.
3. Burke, *Optimal Muscle Performance and Recovery*, 46.
4. Ylinen, *Sports Massage*, 13.
5. Anderson, *Stretching*, 9.
6. Ibid.

## Chapter 13

1. Tedeschi, *Essential Anatomy*, 8.
2. Ibid., 30.
3. Gach, *Acupressure's Potent Points*, 3; and Wildish, *The Book of Ch'i*, 46.
4. Wildish, *The Book of Ch'i*, 49.
5. Gach, *Acupressure's Potent Points*, 5.
6. Wildish, *The Book of Ch'i*, 54; and Gach, *Acupressure's Potent Points*, 5.
7. Tedeschi, *Essential Anatomy*, 42.
8. Ibid.
9. Stux, *Basics of Acupuncture*, 2.
10. Ibid., 1.
11. Ibid., 26.
12. Ibid., 7–8.
13. Ibid.
14. Gach, *Acupressure's Potent Points*, 5.
15. Stux, *Basics of Acupuncture*, 9.
16. Ibid., 30. "Thoren showed that prolonged 'jogging' in spontaneously hypertensive rats produced exactly the same effects as acupuncture (jogging produced analgesia and lowered blood pressure via serotonin and endorphin mechanisms), suggesting that type III muscle afferents may function normally to induce analgesia during severe exercise."
17. Gach, *Acupressure's Potent Points*, 10.
18. Ibid., 10.
19. Ibid., 6, and Tedeschi, *Essential Anatomy*, 46.
20. Tedeschi, *Essential Anatomy*, 46.
21. Ibid.

## Chapter 14

1. Davies, *The Trigger Point Therapy Workbook*, 2.
2. Ibid., 25.
3. Ibid., 3.
4. Ibid., 39.
5. Ibid., 17.

6. Ibid., 37.
7. Ibid., 19.
8. Ibid.
9. Ibid.
10. Ibid., 38–40.
11. Ibid., 38.

## Chapter 15

1. Waterpik makes a number of very effective handheld shower heads with varying degrees of intensely pulsating sprays.
2. To get a feel for the dangers of shrinkage see the *Seinfeld* season five episode "The Hamptons."

## Chapter 17

1. Weil, *Health and Healing*, 236; and Kogler, *Yoga for Athletes*, 11–12.
2. Shaw, *The Little Book of Yoga Breathing*, 19–22.
3. Maher, *An Open Life—Joseph Campbell in Conversation with Michael Toms*, 23.
4. Murphy, *In the Zone*, 153–158; and McGee, *Magical Running*, 101; and Higdon, *Marathon The Ultimate Training Guide*, 183–189.

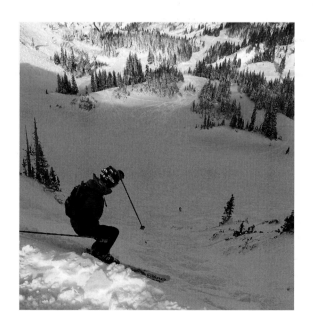

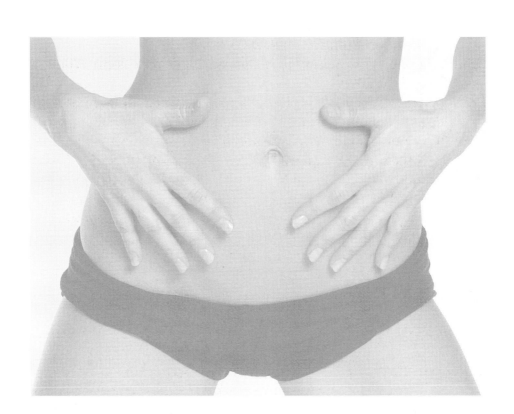

# References

Anderson, Bob, illustrated by Jean Anderson. *Stretching*. Bolinas, CA: Shelter Publications, Inc., 1980.

Armstrong, Lance, with Sally Jenkins. *It's Not About the Bike*. New York: Berkeley Books, 2000.

Ballentine, Rudolph, MD, and Swami Rama. *Science of Breath*. Honesdale, PA: Himalayan Institute Press, 1979.

Benjamin, Patricia J., and Frances M. Tappan. *Tappan's Handbook of Healing Massage Techniques*, 4th Edition. Upper Saddle River, NJ: Pearson Prentice Hall, 2005.

Braun, Stephen. *The Science of Happiness*. New York: John Wiley & Sons, Inc., 2000.

Burke, Edmund R., Ph.D. *Optimal Muscle Performance and Recovery*. New York: Avery Penguin Putnam, 1999.

Calvert, Robert Noah. "Pages from History: The Greek Gymnasium." *Massage Magazine*, (March/April 2005): 172–175.

Clay, James H., and David M. Pounds. *Basic Clinical Massage Therapy: Integrating Anatomy and Treatment*. Philadelphia: Lippincott Williams & Wilkins, 2003.

Cooper, Andrew. *Playing in the Zone*. Boston: Shambhala Publications Inc., 1998.

Davies, Clair. *The Trigger Point Therapy Workbook*. Oakland, CA: New Harbinger Publications, Inc., 2001.

Downing, George. *The Massage Book*. New York: Random House, 1972.

Eisenberg, David M., MD, Roger B. Davis, ScD, Susan L. Ettner, PhD, Scott Appel, MS, Sonja Wilkey, Maria VanRompay, Ronald C. Kessler, PhD. "Trends in Alternative Medicine Use in the United States, 1990–1997." *Journal of the American Medical Association* 280(18) (November 11, 1998): 1569–1575.

Field, Tiffany. *Touch*. Cambridge, MA: MIT Press, 2001.

Field, Tiffany. *Touch Therapy*. Edinburgh: Churchill Livingstone, 2000.

Field, T., N. Grizzle, F. Scafidi, S. Schanberg. "Massage and Relaxation Therapies' Effects on Depressed Adolescent Mothers." *Adolescence* 31 (124) (1996): 903–911.

Field, T., T. Henteleff, M. Hernandez-Reif, E. Martinez, K. Mavunda, C. Kuhn, and S. Schanberg. "Children with Asthma Have Improved Pulmonary Functions after Massage Therapy." *Journal of Pediatrics* 132 (1997): 854–858.

Field, T., G. Ironson, F. Scafidi, T. Nawrocki, A. Goncalves,

I. Burman, J. Pickens, N. Fox, S. Schanberg, and C. Kuhn. "Massage Therapy Reduces Anxiety and Enhances EEG Pattern of Alertness and Math Computations." *International Journal of Neuroscience,* 86 (1996): 197–205.

Gach, Michael Reed. *Acupressure's Potent Points: A Guide to Self-Care for Common Ailments.* New York: Bantam Books, 1990.

Grossberg J.M., and E.F. Alf, Jr. "Interaction with Pet Dogs: Effects on Human Cardiovascular Response." *Journal of the Delta Society* 12 (1985): 20–27.

Hart, S., T. Field, M. Hernandez-Reif, G. Nearing, S. Shaw, S. Schanberg, and C. Kuhn. "Anorexia Nervosa Symptoms Are Reduced by Massage Therapy." *Eating Disorders* 9 (2001): 289–299.

Hernandez-Reif, M., T. Field, J. Dieter, and M. Diego Swerdlow. "Migraine Headaches Are Reduced by Massage Therapy." *International Journal of Neuroscience* 96 (1998): 1–11.

Hernandez-Reif, M., T. Field, S. Leivaldi, et al. (In Press). "University Dance Students Show Increased Range of Motion Following Massage Therapy." *Journal of Dance Medicine & Science Psychology* 24:183–189.

Hernandez-Reif, M., A. Martinez, T. Field, O. Quintero, and S. Hart. "Premenstrual Syndrome Symptoms Are Relieved by Massage Therapy." *Journal of Psychosomatic Obstetrics & Gynecology* 21 (2000): 9–15.

Higdon, Hal. *Marathon The Ultimate Training Guide.* New York: Rodale Press, 1999.

Jarmey, Chris, and John Tindall. *Acupressure for Common Ailments.* New York: Simon & Schuster, 1991.

Johnson, Joan. *The Healing Art of Sports Massage.* New York: Rodale Press, 1995.

Juhan, Dean. *Job's Body,* 3rd edition. Barrytown, NY: Barrytown/Statin Hill Press Inc., 1987.

Kogler, Aladar, Ph.D. *Yoga for Athletes.* St. Paul, MN: Llewellyn Publications, 1995.

Kolata, Gina. "Runner's High? Endorphins? Fiction, Some Scientists Say." *The New York Times,* May 21, 2002.

Kubsch, S.M., T. Neveau, and K. Vandertie. "Effect of Cutaneous Stimulation on Pain Reduction in Emergency Department Patients." *Complementary Therapies in Nursing & Midwifery,* 6 (2000): 25–32.

Kurz, Thomas. *Stretching Scientifically.* Island Pond, VT: Stadion Publishing Company, 1987.

Levinthal, Charles F. *Messengers of Paradise.* New York: Anchor Press Doubleday, 1988.

Leivadi, S., M. Hernandez-Reif, T. Field, M. O'Rourke, S. D'Arienzo, D. Lewis, N. del Pino, S. Schanberg, C. Kuhn. "Massage Therapy and Relaxation Effects on University Dance Students." *Journal of Dance Medicine & Science,* 3 (1999): 108–112.

Madden J., Akil H. Barchas JD, et al. "Stress induced parallel changes in central opioid levels and pain responsiveness in rat." *Nature* 265 (1977): 358–360.

Maher, John A., and Dennie Briggs, Editors. *An Open Life—Joseph Campbell in Conversation with Michael Toms.* New York: Harper & Row Publishers, 1989.

Maxwell-Hudson, Clare. *Complete Massage.* London: DK Publishing, 1999.

Maxwell-Hudson, Clare. *The Complete Book of Massage.* New York: Random House, 1988.

McGee, Bobby. *Magical Running.* Boulder, CO: Bobbysez Publishing, 2000.

Micheli, Lyle J., with Mark Jenkins. *The Sports Medicine Bible.* New York: Quill, HarperCollins Publishers, 2001.

Murphy, Michael, and Rhea A. White. *In the Zone: Transcendent Experience in Sports.* New York: Penguin Arkana, 1978.

Nickel, David J. *Acupressure for Athletes.* New York: Henry Holt and Company, 1984.

Ogal, Hans P. *The Seirin Pictorial Atlas of Acupuncture.* Cambridge, U.K.: Koneman, 2000.

Paine, Tim. *The Complete Guide to Sports Massage.* London: A&C Black, 2000.

Pelé, with Robert L. Fish. *My Life and the Beautiful Game.* Garden City, NY: Doubleday, 1977.

Pert, Candace B., Ph.D. *Molecules of Emotion.* New York: Touchstone Simon & Schuster, 1997.

Richards, K.C. "The Effect of a Back Massage and Relaxation Intervention on Sleep." *American Journal of Critical Care* 7 (4), (1998): 288–299.

Riggs, Art. *Deep Tissue Massage.* Berkeley, CA: North Atlantic Books, 2002.

Serizawa, Katsusuke, MD. *Massage, The Oriental Method.* Tokyo: Japan Publications, 1972.

Shaw, Scott. *The Little Book of Yoga Breathing.* Boston: Weiser Books, 2004.

Shrier, Ian. "Stretching Before Exercise Does Not Reduce the Risk of Local Muscle Injury: A Critical Review of the Clinical and Basic Science Literature." *Clinical Journal of Sport Medicine* Vol. 9, No. 4 (1999): 221–227.

Shrier, Ian. "Myths and Truths of Stretching." *The Physician and Sports Medicine* Vol. 28, No. 8 (2000): 324–325.

Shulman, K.R., and G.E. Jones. "The Effectiveness of Massage Therapy Intervention on Reducing Anxiety in the Workplace." *Journal of Applied Behavioral Science* 32 (1996): 160–173.

Smith, L.L., M.N. Keating, D. Holbert, et al. "The Effects of Athletic Massage on Delayed Onset Muscle Soreness, Creatine Kinase, and Neutrophil Count: a Preliminary Report." *Journal of Orthopaedic & Sports Physical Therapy,* 19 (1994): 93–99.

Stux, Gabriel, and Bruce Pomeranz. *Basics of Acupuncture,* 4th Edition. Berlin: Springer, 1997.

Tedeschi, Marc. *Essential Anatomy.* New York: Weatherhill, 2000.

Teenguarden, Iona Marsaa. *A Complete Guide to Acupressure,* Revised Edition. Tokyo: Japan Publications, Inc., 2002.

Vickers, Andrew. *Massage and Aromatherapy: A Guide for Health Professionals.* London: Chapman & Hall, 1996.

Walters, Lynne. *Kind Touch Massage.* New York: Sterling Publishing Co. Inc., 2002.

Weil, Andrew, MD. *Health and Healing.* Boston: Houghton Mifflin Company, 1998.

Werner, Ruth. *A Massage Therapist's Guide to Pathology*, 2nd Edition. Philadelphia: Lippincott Williams & Walker, 2002.

Wildish, Paul. *The Book of Ch'i.* Boston: Tuttle Publishing, 2000.

Ylinen, Jari, and Mel Cash. *Sports Massage.* London: Ebury Press, 1988.

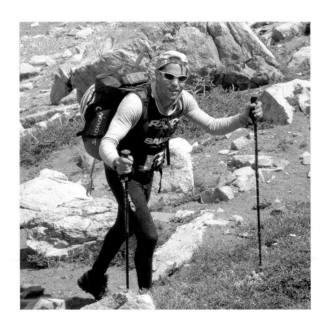

# Index

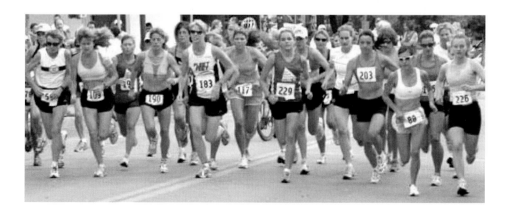

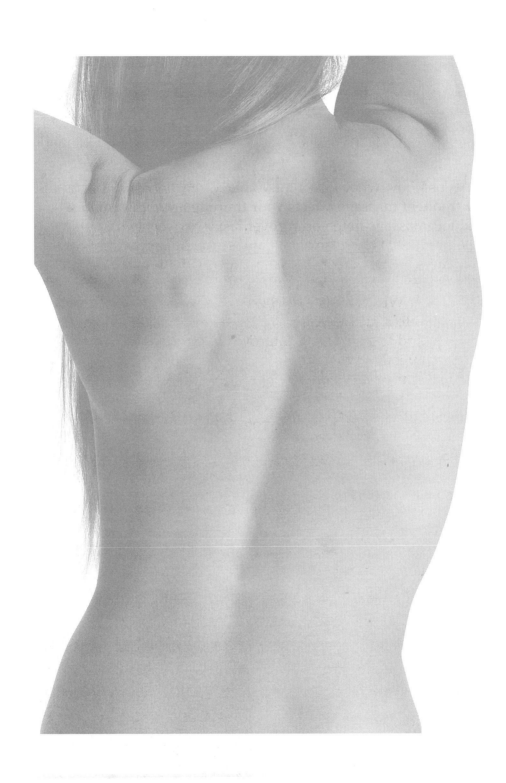

# Afterword

We know that self-massage will help you feel better, and hope it gives you a better understanding of your body, its strengths, and its weaknesses. As you practice self-massage, you're sure to discover many new things about yourself as an athlete. Whatever you find we'd like to hear about it.

Let us know what works for you, and what doesn't. Tell us how frequent massage affects your training and performance. Does self-massage help you recover faster between workouts? Does it reduce your muscle pain and soreness as effectively as research indicates? Does it relieve stress? Does it improve your health? How does it affect your mood? Do massage tools make a difference? Which tools work best? Were you able to turn your bathroom into a spa as easily as the book suggests? Do pressing acupoints and trigger points improve your massage? Is power breathing effective?

Share your findings with other athletes. We'd like to include your ideas in the next edition of this book, and at our website. Please direct your suggestions and thoughts to: SelfMassageForAthletes.com.

As for this book, if you found it helpful, let us know, and pass the word on to your friends, training partners, and teammates. If you noticed things that can be improved upon, let us know that too.

We hope it guides you to a fuller more rewarding athletic life.

Keep in touch.

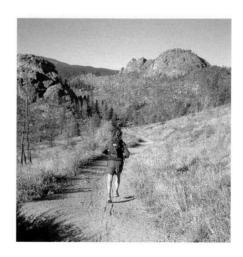

## Contact Us:

For more information about self-massage
For additional copies of this book
To learn more about self-massage tools
For information about our workshops, clinics, and classes
To learn about our team discounts
To share your ideas about self-massage for athletes
We want to hear from you

## SelfMassageForAthletes.com

*Where athletes, massage therapists, and active people of all kinds go to learn more about self-massage*

### Write to Us:

Two Hand Press, LLC
P.O. Box 4236
Boulder, CO 80306

## Keep in Touch

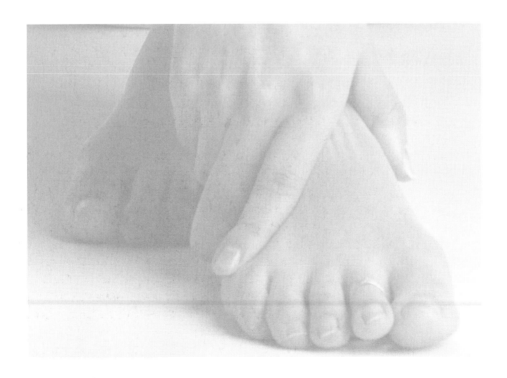